ADVANCE PRAISE

'This book is a vital and timely exploration of a poorly understood and devastating mental illness, and a powerful meditation on the fragility and resilience of selfhood. It will resonate profoundly with all those who question what it means to be ourselves, and what it is to be human.'

Elinor Cleghorn, author of *Unwell Women*

'Nathan Dunne is a writer of such touching sympathies and affinities and generosity and pure gifts of language and mastery of both echoes internal and in the air.'

Cynthia Ozick, author of *The Puttermesser Papers* and *Antiquities*

'Dunne's writing is extraordinary, original and rewarding.'

Robert Cottrell, *BBC Culture*

when nothing feels real

when nothing feels real

A JOURNEY INTO THE MYSTERY ILLNESS OF DEPERSONALISATION

nathan dunne

murdoch books

Sydney | London

Published in 2025 by Murdoch Books, an imprint of Allen & Unwin

Murdoch Books Australia
Cammeraygal Country
83 Alexander Street, Crows Nest NSW 2065
Phone: +61 (0)2 8425 0100
murdochbooks.com.au
info@murdochbooks.com.au

Murdoch Books UK
Ormond House, 26–27 Boswell Street, London WC1N 3JZ
Phone: +44 (0) 20 8785 5995
murdochbooks.co.uk
info@murdochbooks.co.uk

 A catalogue record for this
book is available from the
National Library of Australia

A catalogue record for this book is available from the British Library

ISBN 978 1 76150 077 0

Cover design by George Saad
Typeset by Midland Typesetters
Printed and bound in Australia by the Opus Group

*Murdoch Books acknowledges the Traditional Owners of the Country on which we
live and work. We pay our respects to all Aboriginal and Torres Strait Islander Elders,
past and present.*

10 9 8 7 6 5 4 3 2 1

 The paper in this book is FSC® certified.
FSC® promotes environmentally responsible,
socially beneficial and economically viable
management of the world's forests.

The horrific struggle to establish a human self results in a self whose humanity is inseparable from that horrific struggle. Our endless and impossible journey toward home is in fact our home.

— DAVID FOSTER WALLACE

Note on the Type

———

This book was set in EB Garamond. Designed by Austrian designer Georg Mayr-Duffner in 2011 to be widely and freely available, the fonts are based on types first cut by Claude Garamond (c. 1480-1561), which were later adapted into the Egenolff–Berner specimen (hence 'EB'), first printed in 1592.

Garamond was a pupil of Geoffroy Tory and is believed to have followed the Venetian models, although he introduced a number of important differences, and it is to him that we owe the letter we now know as 'old style.' He gave to his letter a certain elegance and feeling of movement that won their creator an immediate reputation and the patronage of Francis I of France.

Contents

Prologue

It was approaching midnight. Despite London's winter cold, Maria and I decided to go night swimming. I wheeled my bicycle out of the gate and onto the pavement. My bike made a rusty creak as I squared up the frame and put my feet on the pedals, looking ahead at Maria who blew dust off her handlebars. She turned to me with a smile, and a light wind rushed in among the strands of her hair. Her youth was held by the dark, tree shadows dancing across her face.

The streets were shiny with old rain and streetlights. Car tyres and letterboxes passed in a blur. On one lawn a drunk couple staggered through a garden, kicking the flowers. Maria laughed at the sight of them and, sharp as a church bell, she gave a shout of excitement.

Cold air clung to my face. As I rode, it was as if I was merging with the bicycle and the night air, the shifting of my heels joining with the solid frame, its clarity and purpose, dodging parked cars, weaving through rubbish, the jolt of my arse in the seat as I tried to speed up and jump the gutter. All I could think about was the sensation of my body plunging into the cold water. When we turned from Chester Road into Swain's Lane, I felt like we were crossing from an old country into a new world.

Maria and I had met a year earlier, when she was working as an usher at an old theatre called the Greenwich. It was New Year's Eve. The lighting had an uncommon glow, with candles filling the stage. I made a fool of myself asking Maria out, knocking over a tray of drinks in the process. Maria was chiselled and shy. With black hair that marked her Portuguese lineage, she had incredibly sad eyes, as if her ancestors had passed down ancient sorrow. Up close, you could see a deep scar across the bridge of her nose where she had fallen from a swing and broken her nose as a child. On our first proper date, she arrived carrying André Breton's *Nadja*. She dreamed of being an artist. On the book's slip cover she had drawn statues and plane crashes in black pen.

I was in my first year of graduate study at the University of London, and devoted much of my time to researching a conceptual artist called John Latham. Recently deceased, Latham had a long career and produced thousands of paintings, sculptures and performances. After witnessing the sinking of the

German battleship *Bismarck* in World War II, he became haunted by images of drowning soldiers. I loved being a student. It was the greatest joy to immerse myself in the history of art. All that paint, muck and intellect. All that desire for creation. Looking at this art, contemplating its material and structure, made me feel alive. My daily routine was often spent at home, working on my thesis, or at the college library poring over exhibition catalogues and reviews by snarky critics.

Art was one of the reasons I fell so deeply in love with Maria. It was something we shared, spending entire days in conversation about the art we admired and the strange dis-connect between what was written and said about it. Images and articles about exhibitions filled our texts. We kissed on the steps of Tate Britain and the Victoria and Albert Museum, kissed on the lawn outside the Serpentine Gallery, and kissed in front of Botticelli's painting *Venus and Mars* at the National Gallery. After Maria moved in with me, we lay on the floor listening to records and stared up at the ceiling in the dark. When she laughed at some of the bad lyrics, I leaned over and kissed her scar.

Arriving at the edge of Hampstead Heath, we dropped our bikes and made our way up the hill, moving silently between the trees that seemed to lead us towards a secret rustling in the grass. We shed our clothes at the edge of the pond and waded into the shallows. Stars shimmered on the water and a half-moon bobbed in the inky black. It was so cold we saw our breath. Swimming out to the middle, we fingered mosses and reeds, then began diving under the water and coming up in wild leaps, splashing one another in a game. In close, she nuzzled my cheek with her nose and lips, her tenderness seemed to come through my skin and settle for a moment.

Immediately afterwards, something happened.

I was hit with a great force, torn in two, ripped from myself.

I swam frantically towards the bank, trying to reach solid ground. Even though my head stayed above water, it was like a great hand was trying to push me down to the bottom of the pond, where the black mud and the sludge would wrap me up like a mummy.

There were no lights, never were. No doors, no keys, no sound. Only a black cave of suffocation and terror and whirling black dust. My eyes were full of black soot. I couldn't see. I kept reaching up to clear my eyes, but the soot wouldn't stop piling up. The more I cleared the soot away, the more there seemed to be.

I was leaving my body.

Bent over in the shallows, I clutched my chest, trying to hold my sense of self together. There was nothing I could do. I cried, tears streaming. I couldn't stop. My whole face began to shake, my cheeks going into spasms and my nose dripping snot that mixed with the tears to form a sour metal taste on my lips. I continued clutching at my chest and the air, but it was hopeless.

For a moment, everything stopped.

I stared at my wet hands. They were ghostlike, not my own. I had disappeared, and what was left of me was only a shell. I lost my words.

Maria's voice was far away. 'Nathan, Nathan. Can you hear me?'

Naked before her, dripping with water, I said nothing in response. I couldn't. In a single moment, a split second, I had been locked away, condemned to wander in a body that was not my own. All my nerve endings had, like tiny candlewicks, been set alight. A searing pain tightened around my spine. The great hand was squeezing me from behind. Was it day or night? I knew it was after midnight, here, right by the water, but at the same time I doubted my jangled senses.

Slowly, the soot began to clear, and I could see again. Maria's face was a stranger's, just as my body was that of an unfamiliar entity.

The light on the heath was muted, imprisoned in a tomb of mineral rocks.

Finding my words, I said, 'I'm not me.'

'What do you mean?' asked Maria.

'I'm not myself. I'm lost.'

'It's okay, love,' she said, scratching the tip of her tongue with her front teeth. 'It's just very cold, you're probably a bit dizzy.'

I screamed out, a primitive and bloodcurdling sound, a part of me that I'd never accessed before. I wasn't sure it was even my own scream. Maria put her hands on my shoulders.

I turned away and ran into the long grass in chaotic, dizzying steps, picking up speed, weaving between logs and rocks with ferocious energy. My thighs had sharp pains. I staggered into a thin stream of moonlight. Stars began to dot my vision. All the blood in my body poured into my face, piling between my skull and skin.

When I finally stopped running, it felt like I'd been going for miles. But Maria was right there, meaning I couldn't have gone too far. She spoke to me softly for several minutes, leaning in close with a hard look of concern and irritation. I couldn't hear what she said, only muffled sounds.

'Seriously,' I said to Maria, who was, herself, taking deep breaths. 'What the fuck is happening?'

I fished around in my pile of clothes and found my wallet. For years, I had kept a VICTORY 1945 medal inside its plastic pocket, having bought it at a Sunday market because it reminded me of my grandfather, who fought in the Pacific during World War II. While it was a cheap object, it said to me that if my bloodline can survive war, I can survive being out in the streets at peacetime, whatever the trouble. I held the medal in my palm, turning it over and over, pressing it hard into my skin.

The medal weighed me down, and I needed it, a precious worldly anchor in a terrifying new land, one with an entirely new map for sensing and feeling and thinking. I wanted to go back to before the swim, where everything would be as it was.

Maria blinked, very slowly. 'Let's get you out of here.'

1

The Great Hand

Back inside the flat, coats hung, I continued to unravel. My words and thoughts ran away from one another and then circled back, criss-crossing, appearing then disappearing. I had to pretend that I could talk properly, that this voice was really mine, that this façade of skin was really me. But the performance was hard to maintain and took all my energy. I felt that the more I clenched my muscles and stood upright, half-smiling, trying to be normal, the more this strange unreality would be gone from me.

'I'm not imagining it,' I said to Maria.

Her mood shifted from amused tolerance to slight concern. 'Do we have to do this now? You'll feel okay after a good night's sleep.'

'I'm sinking.'

'What?' she fired back. 'Get yourself together.'

'I'm going to die.'

She slid a finger along the polished surface of the table. 'Shut up. Not for ninety years.'

I had a frightening sense of moving towards the bathroom, taps running, and lights being turned on and off. In the bedroom, Maria sat me up against our dishevelled pillows and pulled my ruddy corduroy robe in around my shoulders.

My eyes. They're turning themselves inside out.

Before she turned out the light, Maria folded a number of t-shirts, intent on making them as neat as possible, stacking them in a pile on top of the dresser. Even though I was back at home, in my own bed, I felt worse, dangerously bleak. I was stripped raw, my stomach full of pain. I wanted to be cleaved open.

'Please,' I said, begging the darkness. 'Release me from this. Let me return to my body.'

The noise of a passing train.

I couldn't sleep and got up to have a shower. My feeling of having a split self became more acute. One part of my self was empty: a dusty, windswept space. The second part of my self was in a state of confinement. I felt like a puppet, manipulated by something, or someone, outside my body. As I reached for the hot water tap, the part of me that had split off was watching. I turned around to brush away this feeling of being watched, but my second self stayed behind my back. It was looking at me but I couldn't see it. I had no sense of its form or how this second self was moving me around, only that the awareness of 'me' was now gone.

The feeling of not being me, of having no self, was a radical loss of freedom. The sense of being unfree, of having a part of my self imprisoned, was like the reversal of my life's evolution – the reversal of 'me'.

When I woke the next morning, Maria had already left for work at the graphic design firm, where she sat in meetings surrounded by well-dressed colleagues named Stefan and Annaliese. My first thought was a flicker of hope, that everything was okay, that I was myself again, followed immediately by an overwhelming sense that I was still a puppet, watched and controlled by my second self.

I dressed slowly, shirt first, then underwear, speeding up when I put on colourful socks. With a fire burning up my spine, I began to clean, stripping bed sheets, dusting the dresser, wiping benchtops and walls and light switches and picture frames that housed strange photographs of me from another life. Pausing to stare at them made the fire worse. I raced into the lounge room and put on some loud music, turning it up until the windows shook.

'I am twenty-eight years old,' I said to myself, trying to believe it. 'My name is Nathan Dunne.'

I went to the sideboard, picked up a green vase and began storming about wildly, running into walls, and into the bathroom, where I came to the sight of my strange face in the mirror. Every second, every microsecond, was palpable and vicious. The terrifying slow sense of time wrapped up my nerves, searing my psyche. My face contorted in the mirror. *I'm not me.* I chanted to myself, but couldn't make out what I was saying. And then I heard it: my name. I tried to chant my last name, too, but I couldn't.

I started screaming at my face: a gaping wound. A murderous rage built up in me, a medieval cauldron. *Stop.* Violence surged through me, and in my extreme woundedness and terror at the sight of my face, I hurled the vase.

It smashed and the shards littered the tiles.

I reached for the VICTORY 1945 medal in my pocket, rubbing it. Feeling like I might vomit, I lurched towards the toilet. The medal slipped out of my hand into the drain. I dropped to my knees, pressing my fingers into the grate, frantically reaching for the medal. I grabbed an old silver hairbrush and managed to unsettle the grate, only to find pieces of toilet paper and excrement stuck inside. Flakes broke off and stuck to my hand. The smell was of shit and mushy peas.

'Please, no,' I said, begging the drain, and hitting the hard porcelain of the toilet with my fist. 'Please ...'

The smell rushed at my face. I began to gag, but I didn't pull my hand out, reaching in further and desperately fingering the drain – nothing.

I crawled back out onto the carpet and collapsed onto my side, staring at dust motes, waiting. For what? For my stable sense of self to return. For an evaporation of the distance between the two parts of my self: the release of the part in confinement and the re-embodiment of the fragment left behind.

Amidst the tears, I convinced myself that as long as I kept moving, I would stay alive. *Get up. Do it, now.* I put on my yellow raincoat and black gloves, then made for the front door, where I tried the knob several times before committing. It was snowing. I set out walking along the old path, towards the park, which led up to a set of traffic lights that were changing more rapidly than usual.

I spoke to the part of me in confinement, my second self. 'I think I can see you. Can you see me? I think I can hear you listening to me.'

A flock of nuns walked out the doors of St Gabriel's. One of them picked up a snowball and threw it at the back of another nun. A fight was on. Pockets of excited white breath puffed out between them, and in the rush of the game a nun fell over, her black habit spreading out in the snow. She rolled over onto her back while the others quickly gathered around and pelted her with snowballs, hopping and twisting, throwing their heads back, laughing in full view of the sky.

Was any of this real?

The path was uneven, rising and falling with clumps of snow. I was jittery, full of burning pins and needles. I needed a sanctuary. But I wasn't sure exactly where I was. This place, or another place, this street, or the one over by the post office with the stubborn bollards and garish real estate signs, the one I had walked a thousand times.

'Hey,' I said to myself. 'It's this way.'

'No, it's not.'

'What's wrong with me?'

'You're dying.'

Entering the park, it was deathly quiet. Ferns and frosted thorns sprouted from the undergrowth. Coming to a dense crossing of branches, I surprised a wren. It trembled on its perch, before sailing through several trunks and circling back to the perch, where it stared at me. Its stumpy tail flapped in pert excitement. Something about the freedom of this wren to fly between the snow-covered leaves increased my belief that I was, finally, at the end. I would never be able to return to my stable sense of self. A core part of me would remain lost forever. This excruciating, demonic pain had exhausted me. Every moment, every fresh step in the snow, was torment. The mere presence of this tiny free bird, a creature of heaven, crushed me. I banged my head against the tree trunk, over and over again, and when I looked up, the wren was gone. I had no self. I had no grasp of 'me'. I couldn't go on. The nightmare must end. I had been changed, morphed, destroyed, reborn into an aching shell of skin. I was no longer free.

There was only one way out.

———

I waddled into the bathroom and sat on the edge of the bath, turned the taps on at full blast and rocked my head in my hands, trying to soothe or shock my eyes back to their normal state. Nothing worked. The tiles were littered with shards of the broken vase, and I reached for one, running a finger along its sharp edge. Touching my skin with it, I trembled, looking out into the steam, and for a moment I felt the horror of what I was about to do.

All my notions of myself were shattered. My sense of being, self-confidence, self-worth, the way I understood and processed the world, had been ripped away. I sensed that my feeling of no self had its origin in my mind, but I couldn't make sense of how it related to the devastating physical symptoms. My face had become a foreign object. It wasn't a mask. It was the same face I'd always had. But it no longer *looked* or *felt* like mine. I was a stranger without substance or geography.

My love for Maria was everything. She was the only thing that gave me pause. I had just yesterday believed we would be together forever, have a wedding day, children. But none of those dreams could happen any more, not with this disintegrated, empty me.

Slowly and carefully, I sank the shard into my skin, cutting from my ankles to my knees. The next cuts were across my shoulders, running behind my neck. I put the shard in my mouth, where it cut my gums and tongue and warm blood began to drip down my chin.

Staring at the cuts on my legs, they were clean – for a moment – and then, slowly, beneath the water, blood clouded the bath.

How could I call out to my body and say, 'Here, is this you?' There was nothing I could do, no willing of the body itself, no particular action, no single vine out of the cave, nothing to cling to. There was no way to grasp my self any more, no tools to put the two parts back together and stand up and say, 'I am me.'

I peed in the water, warmth spreading, and for a moment it brought back a sense of clarity, a granite belief that for some reason I should stay alive. Scrambling around for my phone,

I saw that it was on its last bar, blinking red. I called Maria, saying something at high pitch, saying enough.

By the time the sirens arrived, I had crawled out of the bath and into bed. The ambulance team hovered over me in the room, uniforms blurring into one, and I heard the quick tear of bandage strips as a woman's hard voice asked me my name. 'Tell me who you are.'

She slapped my face repeatedly, and everything went white.

———

'Mr Dunne?' A voice came out of the darkness. 'Can you sit up a little higher for me?' It was a blue man, narrow-shouldered, long legs. His eyes were wide and penetrating, but veiled, as if he'd been trained to look at me without looking in. His small mouth was a serious line, and all of his fingernails had been bitten to the quick.

'Mr Dunne ...' The tone was mildly threatening; a schoolmaster who'd spent years trying to teach Latin. 'The sedative we gave you should be wearing off. I know you've had a horrible time, but you're safe here now.'

I fingered the bandages on my legs. 'What's wrong with me?'

Beneath his blue coat, he wore a pair of sleek patent-leather shoes. 'Don't cry, son.'

The man helped me out of bed, walking me slowly down a long corridor into a side room. There was a row of thin, adjustable lights, trolleys propped against the walls, and a framed photograph of clouds that sat harmlessly by the soap dispenser.

'Hiya, Tom,' said the blue man in a deep, rich voice.

I was handed off to a shorter man who must have been the ophthalmologist. He wore a plastic cap and spoke gently about eye diseases and vision disorders, guiding me towards a strange goggle machine, which he called 'the instrument'. Soon, I clamped up in horrible pain. I was in another room. Someone must have said 'brain scan' or 'MRI' and my mouth became so dry I could feel every movement of my tongue as it probed the cuts on my gums. The machine bore down on me in terrifying shapes, and the rhythm of its beeps had the on/off throb of $+ - + - + -$, the beat that rides the heart. In the half-light there was a low swell of voices and the sound of pens being dropped into a cast-iron mug.

Dread clawed at the pit of my stomach.

'This won't take long at all,' said a repulsive voice.

On my back, alone in the machine, I thought of all the work I was neglecting. How would I ever be able to get back to it? And did I even want to? It seemed irrelevant, even ridiculous. I couldn't possibly think about the soldiers, not any more. And my finances, already dire, would dry up if I didn't get it together. The only income I had was from an almost depleted student loan and what I could make as a freelance copywriter, which wasn't much.

Although my sense of self was gone, I told myself: 'This mind is still my own.' I hoped it was.

Once I left the machine and was able to amble around the ward – rooms groaning with the noise of television cowboys, others smelling of cough mixture and faeces – a woman in gloves appeared in front of me.

'There's someone here for you. She's waiting for you in the cafe.'

Maria at a round table, hands folded in her lap. When she saw my dishevelled state she began to cry, but she didn't turn her head away.

I cried too. It felt like I'd never be able to stop.

'What's happened to you?'

'I'm sorry ...'

She stroked my brow with cool fingers, like a young mother trying to tell if her child has a fever. 'I didn't know things were so bad.'

'I didn't know either. It all happened so quickly.'

She cuddled against me silently, kissing my hands several times, before catching herself and pulling back.

'Things will get better,' I said, my voice straining, trying to sound convincing.

'The house is a mess. Are you ready to talk to me?'

'I can't explain. It's like I am dead, like I'm not really here with you now.'

Her bony knees tilted together under the table. 'Why did you break the vase?'

'I didn't recognise myself any more. I left my body.'

'What did the doctors say?'

'They're going to call me with some results this week.'

Her face was stiff and puzzled. 'Why is it such a mystery? Are you depressed?'

On the table next to us there was the low rasping sound of a grandmother turning the pages of a newspaper. She was enjoying her Coke.

'I brought you a change of clothes,' said Maria, gesturing to a white shopping bag at her side.

I pulled out the shirt, a baggy Hawaiian that I'd only ever worn once on a foolish day trip to Brighton.

'I thought the colour would make you happy, make you feel better.'

———

That evening we ate chicken and baked potatoes and salad with too much balsamic dressing. There was no conversation. The red digits on the clock said 8:16. I felt the return of some energy, and after we were done, while Maria loaded the dishwasher, I scraped the chicken bones and soiled napkins into a big black garbage bag. She moved heavily on the linoleum, folding tea towels. I managed to smile for her, and she came to lift up my t-shirt, running her fingers gently over my bandages, before scratching my back.

'Maybe you had a stroke.' Her voice was clipped and subtly condescending. 'A minor one, it could be.'

'Maybe.'

'We should have never gone swimming. It was a bad idea.'

I pulled on her pyjama sleeve. 'I love you.'

She shifted away and put her hands in the sink, fishing around in the cutlery. 'You might be right.'

'What does that mean? *You might be right.*'

Shaking her head. 'This is too difficult.'

A sharp, fiery pain rose up my spine. 'I need you to be here for me right now.'

'Thank you for helping with the garbage. I know you must be exhausted.'

'Maria.'

'I can't see you like this.'

I reached again for her sleeve.

She went to bed early and I typed *minor stroke* into a search engine, immediately regretting it. My nerves were coarse and brutal. Among the statistics and helplines and alarming personal testimonies, I came across several articles that suggested we are all dying of cancer. All the time. Sad click after sad click, articles and forums and feeds, scrolling endlessly in an effort to distract from the pain in my spine, to find out what was wrong. Oh, and WebMD, always terrifying, belittling, the fire that never goes out.

It's brain disease, no it's heart disease; it's depression, the worse kind, clinical, the deepest black, no one returns from this kind; it's schizophrenia, of course it is, the delusions, the voices, the seasons all have one name; it's cataracts, lung disease, bowel cancer – yes – probably got a month. No, that's ridiculous: maybe it's colorectal cancer or bladder cancer or kidney cancer, the data, deadly, the stats, bad cells, common in men, chances extremely high, yes, it's some type of cancer, the hourglass in my lap; it's fibromyalgia, chronic fatigue, diabetes, body dysmorphia, capgras delusion, Diogenes syndrome, Huntington's disease, transient global amnesia, amaurosis fugax, encephalitis, Joubert syndrome, Creutzfeldt–Jakob disease, Wolfram syndrome, dystonia, thalassemia, dysthymia, early dementia, sounds right, can't think, can't remember; cirrhosis, hepatitis; no it's bipolar, splitting open, the trap door, it has to be, this is it, the highs, the lows, mania. Am I bipolar? What the fuck is this? No, it has to be brain cancer.

It's hard to describe my bewildering panic at not knowing what was wrong with me when something was so deeply wrong with me. I was reduced to the status of a child, helpless and stumbling, trying desperately to reach solid ground. I'd lurch between denial, 'It's nothing,' and catastrophe, 'This is the end.' The panic was so great that I'd descend into clichés: *One day at a time, This is not how my story will end, The sun will always rise in the morning.* When I was of a healthy body and mind, I might have dismissed these as Hallmark card platitudes. But now these clichés held universal truths of resilience and survival.

Even when coming down with a common cold, you never really know how bad it will be, whether you'll have a chest cough or a dry cough, how many days you might need to take off work, whether you'll need to go to the doctor, how much that will cost, whether you'll be able to care for your children or be able to sleep. But now, when the core of my existence, my self, that centre that held me together, was no longer in place, it was like a razor-sharp sword had been jammed down my spine, breaking me in half, casting an essential part of me into a violent storm.

I thought of the VICTORY 1945 medal and how I used to hold it in my hand for comfort, how I would turn it over and press it into my skin, thinking of my grandfather. I wanted to feel its anchor again, the rough texture of its age and the scent of its cheap metal, the way it promised an extension of me. But it was gone now, fallen through the grate into the dark, far beneath me – lost forever.

If I chose to keep living it would always be like this, trying hopelessly to balance on a tiny rock, on this crumbling, unsteady planet. My life was nothing but waiting for the avalanche of hell to bury me in fire. 'Fuck you! I will survive!' They were stupid words. Inside my heart, I knew I wouldn't survive. Soon, I'd be gone from this earth. Every thought I'd ever had about not being good enough, a fraud and a coward and a second-rate lost cause and having a defective brain and bad genes and not being able to do anything right out here in a cruel world of broken humanity, those thoughts had been right. They had led me to this moment of total abandonment and abject loneliness, of living in an uninhabited body. The pain would never cease. No one cared, *not really*. Maybe Maria did, but how long could she tolerate me in this state? No one would be truly there for me and give me the endless, selfless love I desperately needed. I was alone, a petrified little boy. Each minute that passed pressed tighter on me, the great hand holding me down, drowning me, making sure I knew that there was nothing I could do.

I fought with everything I had to stay off the balcony. But I was completely in the grip of the illness. I wanted to die ferociously and instantly. It was urgent. Slam on the asphalt and have my guts smashed upwards against my broken ribs and cracked neck and torn shoulders, nothing left of me but a smear of organs and bones. Only after my physical body had been obliterated would this chamber of hell burst open. Only then would the world stop being a burden and I a burden to it.

I looked down at my withering hands, full of spots and lines. My hands were those of a ghost. They were not my own.

2

The Possibles

It would take me some time, a lot of time, before I understood what was happening to me: I was experiencing depersonalisation. Its onset provoked a profound loss of identity. Like many with the illness, my response was to say, 'I'm not me,' 'I have no self' and 'I am no one.' This was an attempt to describe the feeling of a severe dissociative state, the onset of mental illness, pure terror. My identity had always been intrinsically tied up with my body, fundamental to my self-consciousness. When I looked in the mirror, I'd say, 'I'm this tall, this heavy. I have this mole, this chin. I have these eyes, these hands.' But with depersonalisation, being in its vice meant a terrifying challenge to long-held assumptions about my existence – the notion of 'me'. The name of the illness itself described my personhood being emptied out.

According to research conducted by the Pew Research Center in Washington, DC, the global DSM-5 Research Group and a team of international doctors who specialise in depersonalisation, it is estimated that more than 75 million people worldwide suffer from the illness. In the United States, it affects 2 per cent of the population – 6.4 million. In Britain, it's 1.3 million. In Australia, this would extrapolate to about 500,000.

My feeling of being locked into an absence of identity, the feeling of no self, meant that I had no choice but to remain outside my body as a detached observer. For me, the vantage point of this detachment felt like being in a specific place, a damp black box. But for other patients, like Amanda, a 43-year-old office assistant, 'It is as if the real me is taken out and put on a shelf or stored somewhere.' Alex, a merchant marine from New York, says: 'It was something like waking up to find that you're in a coffin, buried alive. Only the coffin is your body, your very existence.'

Being depersonalised felt like my mind was working outside my body. It was impossible to think clearly because the part of me in confinement, my second self, was the one organising and constructing my thoughts. My obsessive desire for suicide felt like that of a stranger. If I did jump,

I wasn't sure it would be me who leapt. At first, although I was shut off from myself, I could still access memories about who I once was, or *thought* I was. But this sense of an out-of-place mind created a breakdown in those memories. I processed time differently, and sometimes it appeared to stop altogether, like when I first came out of the Hampstead pond. My internal clock sped up, resulting in regular, geophysical time becoming slow – or freezing. Minutes seemed like hours. The recollection of my life lasted only a few seconds.

The illness does strange things to once-vivid memories. They become dislocated, feel like fictions. Sometimes, too, they *are* fictions, projections from a fragment of the past into the present or future. I tried to hold onto a sense of time as memories – especially happy ones – appeared and disappeared without a clear pattern. But feeling like a robot meant that while I could recall a memory, it didn't have the same emotion associated with it, which led me to question whether the event that caused the memory ever happened at all. My memory palace, once held up by sturdy brick and filled with long, well-lit corridors, was on fire. In its wake, a litter of burnt-out and broken imagery. Death felt like the next step in my ever-increasing dissociation.

At first, I called friends and family, trying to explain my symptoms and state of mind when I had clear, lucid bursts.

But I could never find the right words. The problem felt impossible: how to convey an experience of my sense of self having disappeared? I had no linguistic framework for the self in confinement, no elevator pitch for easy comprehension. Soon I gave up, turning my phone off and shoving it away in my bottom drawer among handkerchiefs and figurines. Once I got the all clear from my eye test and MRI, I searched medical journals for clues and stayed up late pondering rare diseases, compiling a word document I saved as 'The Possibles'. Each page of the document was split into four columns. 1/ Psychological 2/ Neurological 3/ Optical 4/ Related Unknowns. It grew daily, like bacteria in a petri dish, multiplying.

'The Possibles' became my sick-boy bible, where I checked and cross-checked symptoms and statistics and prevalence in men of my age. Rearranging the document was like prodding a wild animal. I'd move one disease into a new column, or onto a new page, and it would immediately lash out, more alive in me than ever. I was constantly rating them. Bipolar disorder would get 8/10, then I'd bump it down to 6/10. Wolfram syndrome would be flying steady at 3/10, only to abruptly climb up to a bewildering 7/10. I'd print the document out, underlining symptoms with fat blue lines and scrawling notes to myself across the top of the pages in turquoise letters. Things like: *Blood thing probable, but check page 7. Could be muscular and optical combined, see page 14.*

I also set myself a schoolboy exercise in a footnote.

> Here is the space. Write the answer in it.
> YOU HAVE ....
> Do it with a clear black pen. Again.
> YOU HAVE ....
> Make the letters stand out so that you can always see the answer and remember it for the doctors. If you can write it down there will be no more searching, only clarity.
> Do it. Write it. The answer. No smudges.

Every morning I dragged myself to the screen, blinking at the words I'd pasted and highlighted the night before, only to find myself ever more confused, an ant in an enemy swarm. I was getting nowhere, and the lack of knowledge felt like a seeping wound.

When I was growing up, my mind was always my most reliable companion, my loyal interlocutor, stocked full of things to make me laugh and hold my interest. As an adolescent I found this essential, where my daydreams became time travel. If I was stuck among boring relatives on Christmas Day, I found I could flit out a half-open window and walk down a dusty lane with Flannery O'Connor in the American south;

if I was being lectured about the consequences of poor maths scores by a surly tutor, I slipped out of my chair and joined a team of mountaineers climbing Everest. I trusted my mind completely, and I felt it would always be there to hold me up and rescue me.

Now, in a shocking turn, I was betrayed. My mind called me cruel names, drew out my weaknesses and vulnerabilities, one sin after another paraded in front of me. I was going to hell. Soon I would die, likely by my own hand, and be cast down into the devil's fire. This fire was forever, my mind told me, echoing St Augustine, who wrote that a covenant had been made 'with the devil to darken the spirit and to confine man in the bonds of hell'. *This fire was made for you, it burns for you, waiting to consume your filthy soul. Not long now, you don't have long.*

––––––

I wanted to immerse myself in student life, to have lunch at the Russian cafe near the British Library, scour the footnotes of my thesis, gossip with friends, and browse for new art titles in the bookshops on Charing Cross Road. But since I was incapable of thinking of much else besides death, I was drawn, instead, to the stillness of the local cemetery. It was the only place where my thoughts felt quieter. I carried a tartan blanket with me and lay it over the headstones. I was concerned for the dead, wanted to keep them warm. Sitting cross-legged, I talked to them and cried and ran my hands through the earth, smelling the old soil between my fingers. Curl up with us, I heard them say. But it wasn't the dead talking. They couldn't talk. They were dead. It was my mind, my second self in confinement. I knocked loudly on their tombstones, scraping my knuckles. I said their names amid the towering weeds and wondered who their parents were and what their painful sorry lives – like all lives – were like. I wondered about their final moments, how they died. Would my death be like their deaths?

I called an old friend, Davika, who lived in LA, and while it was a balm to hear her sunny voice and talk about the past, our physical distance was too great. I missed her so much and needed us to sit face to face, to find a bar somewhere in Costa Mesa full of deep leather and heavy glassware where we could talk all night, breathing the same air. After I hung up, I felt the ache of a friend too far away to be of any real help. So I tried desperately to work. I longed for the smell of the college library and the humming quiet of the reading room, hours where I could indulge in thorny sentences and worry about John Latham's paintings.

But I couldn't face the library. Reading was impossible there, and to my intense frustration, in my flat too. Short, simple sentences were suddenly beyond me. The ones I managed to read were immediately stricken from my mind. I was overcome with thinking about drowning soldiers in World War II. I couldn't escape them. My eyes were heavy, forever trying to close. I was used to racing through books, marking pages, typing them up, arguing with them. Now the soldiers were flailing in every paragraph. In my boiling anger, I kicked hardbacks across the room, swearing at them, before staring in shock at their soiled spines, wondering how I'd been so callous.

Audiobooks, mercifully, remained within my grasp, and I fell into them with a great thirst. I listened to Alan Bennett, playwright and famous drizzler, reading his 1980s diaries and became transfixed by an entry about a drowned man. The passage was shattering: 'The water is rising. As he's going down, he slips into a narrow gully. Though he's roped up, the force of the torrent is too much for his companions. As they struggle to pull him out, his light still shining in the water, he drowns.'

I replayed it again and again. Weeping. It was as if this man was me. I found other audiobooks a source of profound transportation and beauty. I must have listened to Richard Burton reading Dylan Thomas's *Under Milk Wood* thousands of times. It also had a cast of drowned men, but because the characters were so funny it rarely troubled me. The recording took me not only to a seaside town in Wales, but to a state of mind that was rich and calm, reined in by absolute pleasure.

But this calm never lasted.

My dark pain was ever-replenishing, my vision disintegrating. Everything was in a dolly zoom, objects foggy, distorted, in pieces. I was acutely *inside* my consciousness, *inside* the part of my self in confinement; I couldn't slip its hold on me.

In my physical weakness, I raged at my entrapment. I promised myself that if I ever got better, I would do whatever it took to conform to the norms of my cousins and neighbours. Watch *Big Brother*? No problem. Get into beetroot salad? Definitely. Listen to the middling tunes of *X-Factor* winners? Sure. Join a team of office workers training to climb Mount Kilimanjaro? Absolutely. Agree with the florist about the wonderful smell of the begonias? One hundred per cent. I wanted the power of control, and so in my faltering head, I conformed, ready to smile earnestly while I accelerated with capitalism and told everyone in the line at Starbucks that their babies were the most beautiful things in the world.

But I wasn't well enough to conform. I had little choice but to go back to 'The Possibles'. Again, I dived into columns of brain cancer and dystonia and Quinquaud's, drawing straight lines between diseases in the document with a plastic ruler. I seemed to have all the symptoms. Never-ending fatigue, unexplained weight loss, brown urine, patchy scalp, impaired vision, arrhythmia, agoraphobia, numbness, feeling of deadness, weird cramps and muscle contractions, bloated ankles, persistent shudders, persistent crying, blackouts. Did it mean I had all these illnesses? Which one was it?

It wasn't just the encyclopedia of illnesses online, but crucially the people on forums discussing them. Here were a thousand lonely tunnels, fomenting with pain. The broken and rejected were everywhere, tiny markings of twitchy names and unbridled fear.

The strangest days were when I felt slightly better. Without warning, I woke with a clearer sense of my body, and renewed energy. The dark pain was dimmed and the fire in my spine was reduced to a dull ache. Breakfast was joyful, crunchy. On one of these days, over a proper helping of muesli, one I could keep down, Maria suggested we wander across to the Serpentine Gallery to see an exhibition and walk the gardens. We took a picnic basket of apples and sourdough and Pepsi and talked about the baby names we liked for a future when everything was upright again – nothing sideways, no more shattered vases. Maria laid out the newspaper and I scanned the sports section, delighted by photographs of footballers in shiny boots.

Even on these days, the illness lingered. It never truly left. Instead, it lay in wait, ready to flare up again and remind me that my brief moments of living in the present and feeling a part of the world were only temporary. Soon, it would return in full force.

And by early spring, it had. The core of me vanished, my stable sense of self once again split. It had now been three months since the onset, and I understood that there were no soft corners. On the good days, even in my hope they might last, I understood the dark pain would always return.

I questioned myself: Isn't there some universal law that says I have the right to go back? Don't I have a right to live in the place where I came from? My former self is still me. My self might be getting smaller in the rear-view mirror, but surely I can reverse, come up close to my former self and make it present again, open the door and wrench it back in?

While I could see myself move, I didn't feel like I was *there* with the movements. Hence the robot feeling and the accompanying terror. My feet would move ahead on the pavement, but they moved on their own, and yet often in excruciating pain. Standing in front of the mirror, something I now tried to avoid, my facial expressions, which had once revealed emotion – the blink of my eyes, the twitch of my lips – were now completely unreal.

I heard my voice as machine-like, generated not from my diaphragm, lungs and throat, but from some alien apparatus outside my body. This is an extremely distressing, yet common, symptom of depersonalisation. The disruption in the brain's ability to integrate sensory and emotional information causes a profound shift in self-awareness. As a result, the perception of one's own voice is altered too. Instead of a stable, external voice, the illness provokes a range of internal voices, which are critical, confused and philosophical. I desperately longed to find my lost voice, reverse time until I found it again.

Who am I? Where am I? Why can't I hear my voice as my own?

One morning I found that my document of 'The Possibles' was missing. I couldn't find it on my laptop, and in a wild panic I backed up my computer and scrolled through endless files searching for it. When I eventually did locate the document, it was empty. All that work, all those hours of potential knowledge, had vanished because of a digital error. I phoned helplines and watched YouTube clips on file recovery, but they all said it was hopeless. There was no 'Undo' function with something like this. Shortly after lunch, Maria walked in to find me staring at the blank screen. I'd never told her about 'The Possibles', although she knew I was in some sort of internet death spiral. She sat across from me on a stool, staring, phone in hand, with her legs tightly crossed and her elbows on the knee of one leg.

Then she began to shout. 'Are you fucking listening to me?'

I hadn't been aware of her voice.

'See a doctor tomorrow or else I'm going to leave you.'

———

Our word 'diagnosis' comes from the Greek *diagignōskein*, meaning 'to discern, to recognise', literally 'to know apart from another'. To be without a diagnosis is to be in a wordless place, without comfort or recognition. But when we have the language for a specific illness, it gives our pain a structure beyond mere symptoms. It grants a shape to the pain and helplessness, implying an end point to suffering. Even with a chronic illness that spans decades, to have a diagnosis is to have the world of medicine on alert for answers. Diagnosis is hope.

It also marks us out from others. On the one hand, it allows entrance into a community of sufferers; on the other, it distances us from the larger group of those without the illness. Those who are healthy, and those with another condition. When we are diagnosed, it not only renders the illness visible, but gives the patient and doctor a pathway for treatment. Even if treatment options are scant and experimental, it's infinitely better than being lost, not having a guide. Which is why misdiagnosis is incredibly common. The hunger is so great for the patient to be lifted out of the wordless place into knowledge that the clinic often gets it wrong, diverting the path to treatment, delaying knowledge that would truly illuminate and cure.

I'd been reluctant to go to the doctor. Without having more than a vague description of my symptoms, I didn't trust a clinic to offer the right help. I needed better words. Ideally, a doctor should have been able to sit with me and locate the illness, but my experience in the hospital had convinced me that being in a clinical setting wasn't enough. Instead, all on my own, I'd turned my drive for academic research into the pursuit of a medical mystery, where the stakes felt like life and death. And I knew that they were.

But the following day, with Maria's ultimatum, I went. The doctor was a man whose ruddy complexion and loose cheeks suggested a love for liquor. His line of work meant the close examination of countless failing bodies, and, as a result, he was beginning to morph into a blob himself. Balding, bad teeth, one rogue ear, and all with a polite and perfectly educated voice.

'What seems to be the trouble?'

He listened impatiently while I told him about the stress of graduate school, being haunted by drowned soldiers, of intermittent work, little money, the totally absorbing and complicated love I had for Maria (would she always love me?), the uncertainty and confusion about my future. I told him I was scared of losing my energy, my clarity of thought and my precious spontaneity. And finally, I said, 'It's as if I'm invisible.'

He nodded. Not in recognition, but bewilderment. 'Okay.'

My voice grew feeble, throaty. 'It's as if I'm unreal, like I have disintegrated, like I'm not really here talking to you, and I have a dark pain that won't leave. It only gets worse.'

'Where's the pain? I don't think I understand.'

I tried to hold the line. 'It's as if I am trapped in a box above my head, and I'm looking down wondering whose body this is.'

'Tell me about this box. Is there anything inside it?'

'Black water.'

What a silly idea, said his face. 'And you are inside it, with the black water?'

'Yes.'

'Do you hear any voices?'

I hesitated. 'No, I don't think so.'

'You don't *think* so?'

Scratching my cheek. 'It's more like pure terror, like I'm about to die.'

Maybe I could have tried simple words like *sick, very sick, broken*. Or maybe *locked out, locked away, buried*. Or shadow words like *double, copy, twin*. Or *empty, hollow, void*. Or crazy words like *unmoored, undead, zombie*. Or *submerged, swallowed, drowning*. Or lost words like *vanished, missing, disappeared*. Or maybe I could have just told him about the great hand and that my body was *under the hill inside the great earth*. No words were accurate enough, and there was a real consequence to this, because if I could only have found the right ones the doctor might have seen the puzzle.

Language is often at the heart of misdiagnosis. When speaking with doctors, people with depersonalisation often describe their symptoms with caution, like swimmers testing the water before a dive. How much should I reveal so I can get the right help? How do I prove that I am aware of reality – known as intact 'reality testing' – when my symptoms sound like those of a psychotic? The phrases and words that I used, 'It's as if I'm invisible' and 'unreal', were misunderstood. When I said, 'I have a dark pain that won't leave,' it's easy to see, in retrospect, how it could be interpreted as depression. 'It's as if I am trapped in a box above my head' is a strange, obtuse description for an illness, but it sounds as much like a cognitive complaint as an experiential one referring to a dissociative state. A further complication arises when patients with other mystery maladies that share symptoms with depersonalisation – like dystonia, Guillain-Barré syndrome and Creutzfeldt–Jakob disease – also describe their complaints in general terms.

With the confusion over the language of depersonalisation, my doctor failed to ask relevant screening questions during the assessment, which led to non-detection. He was more interested in locating the pain in my body, which he presumed was more easily tested, measured and understood, than assessing my apparent invisibility.

Even if he had suspected depersonalisation, there is a chance of what in epidemiological literature is called the 'clinician's illusion'. This is a bias based on a particular subgroup of patients. Given that distress levels in depersonalised patients vary along a spectrum, the doctor will tend to assume yours is lower on the spectrum – not very serious – because the most common experience of the condition is transient, not chronic.

Before the onset of my illness, I'd had, like many people, a transient experience of depersonalisation symptoms. On occasion, I'd suddenly observe my own behaviour and be surprised. Driving home in my old Mitsubishi, I'd wonder how I got there, feeling that I was navigating on autopilot. Or while eating a delicious meal (often penne arrabbiata), I'd become immersed and declare, 'I can't believe I ate the whole thing!' When I was thirteen, my baseball team won a local competition and after accepting the trophy, I told my parents, 'When the crowd cheered, I felt like it was happening to somebody else.'

These fleeting moments of being estranged from myself were completely normal, and my sense of identity and selfhood were rapidly restored. In the general population, 50–70 per cent of people report experiencing transient depersonalisation symptoms. My own symptoms were now intransient. They were chronic. But my doctor couldn't see this. Because I couldn't speak it. Still, my diagnosis was swift: anxiety-related depression. He told me it was simply 'the black dog, very common'. He wrote me a script for some expensive blue pills, an SNRI called duloxetine, and said to give it six weeks. 'It'll be like the terror never existed.'

In the moment, in that squalid little office, I was happy. I had finally, finally, finally arrived, crawled out of the black tunnel onto the plain of a new day. Nothing would be the same. I would be free. This was the moment I had dreamed of on countless sleepless nights when I was on the brink of death, where every fibre of me was on fire, where I was moments from leaping onto the asphalt. It was real. I had my answer. No more time on the high balcony, no more fingering the matchboxes and old ropes, no more smashed vases.

But amid the relief, I also felt that my sickness would now be understood as limiting the scope of my life, that it might quarantine me into a category from which I'd never escape.

Watching people pass by out the window, I wanted them to take me into their healthy lives of yoga and green juice, towards brightly lit homes with well-groomed puppies called Rex and Savannah. *Take me away into a new life!*

———

The blue pills gave me horrific side effects – stomach and neck cramps, heartburn, then a heavy bout of vomiting, which lasted for days. My jaw became impossibly stiff. I sweated profusely and lost my appetite. Worst of all, I grew even more exhausted, legs tangled on the lounge. I spent long afternoons listening to bebop, wrapped up in a scarf, and would pick long broken hairs from an old comb and wind them slowly around my finger.

One night when I couldn't sleep, north of 3 am, Maria restless beside me, I got up to make a cup of black tea. Surrounded by pans full of greasy water in the kitchen, holding the tea in my hands, I was overcome with the desire to have a shower. It had been weeks since my last one. I dreaded the wet stall, and yet, finally, stepped inside it with my tea.

As the water flowed from the cheap showerhead, I sipped my tea, and my mind worked itself into a wild storm. I spilt the tea, soaped the same patch above the elbow again and again, time dissolving into endless terrifying thoughts about the night ahead. *I will never be whole. I have to jump. There's no way out.* I was inside the storm, right at the heart of it, at the whirling centre of my terror and pain. I banged my skull on the tiles, banged it again and again. I smashed the mug, tearing the skin from my knuckles, the boiling tea spilling over my feet. And it was only with all the howling that I came to feel, deeply and intuitively, that I'd been misdiagnosed.

———

When I first presented at the clinic, it was more likely than not I would be misdiagnosed. But we don't go to a doctor expecting that; we go for exactly the opposite experience, and when they give us that golden name, something to hold onto, we hold on fast. As I did. At first. Based on data from the National Health Service (NHS) in the UK, an accurate diagnosis for depersonalisation typically takes between eight and twelve years, a shocking statistic. The long wait occurs because doctors are trained to be sceptical of potential outlying diseases, where the most obvious reason for the complaint is usually the right one. Doctors needn't waste time looking for mysterious reasons for the common cold or ankle sprain. But with an illness like depersonalisation, which is easily mistaken for depression, patients like me are misdiagnosed and wait years, through trial and error, for an accurate diagnosis.

There is also a strong belief among clinicians that depersonalisation is extremely rare – an obscurity found only in textbooks, not patients. Many are unaware of how prevalent it is. My doctor's bewildered look and patronising tone suggested ignorance rather than curiosity. But the problem isn't simply a lack of training in dissociative disorders during medical school; it is enshrined at institutional and government level. In the US, depersonalisation is classified as rare by the National Organization for Rare Disorders (NORD). The National Institutes of Health (NIH) also defines a rare disease as one affecting fewer than 200,000 people. Recent studies show that depersonalisation affects at *least* 1 per cent of the population, which far exceeds this threshold.

If we can change this designation of 'rare', it would be a major step towards improving awareness among clinicians in the US, and would reduce the high rates of misdiagnosis. There is a precedent for change, which makes me hopeful. The ICD-11, a medical classification list by the World Health Organization, which had previously classed the disease as 'a rare disorder', was updated in 2019 to more accurately reflect the data. There is no reason why NORD and the NIH cannot follow suit.

During a stretch of warm summer days over the next month, I threw myself at clinics across the city:

— Dr T suggested I might have body dysmorphia or Asperger's.

— Dr M, who wore Chanel No. 5, thought it was seasonal affective disorder.

— Dr P said it was most likely I was on the lower spectrum of bipolar I.

— Dr S wore soft shoes and was overly friendly but had no idea and took my money anyway.

— Dr K seemed convinced it was the result of a cerebral oedema, aka swelling in the brain.

— Dr R spoke about the mystery illness Guillain-Barré syndrome, which causes dissociative symptoms.

— Dr A suggested it was the result of a childhood trauma I couldn't remember.

— Dr J had long fingernails and said woolly things about evolutionary biology and the limits of medicine.

I took countless more tests, sat in basement rooms with tall plants and, in one office at the end of the Thames, drew the outline of my body in crayon while intoning *ommm*. Most of the doctors were well meaning, but in the end they, too, became medical sleuths, guessing and guessing and guessing.

———

'Why are you crying?' Maria said, walking into the kitchen.

I became aware of the dampness on my cheeks. 'I think I'm going blind.'

'The boy who couldn't see,' she said.

It felt cruel. 'Why are you being like that?'

She stared at me in silent frustration, her spidery hand over one eye. 'It's been going on too long and you're just getting worse. If you need any evidence, look around: *you are baking a cake.'*

I'd never baked a cake before. That's what I was crying about. I'd taken it out of the oven, and it was a horrible mess. But now, worse than its brown and cratered blob, I saw something else: a suitcase by her side.

'I can't help you,' she said, 'if you won't help yourself.'

'Got any other clichés for me?'

'Fuck you, I've been here for you.'

I gnawed on the ragged cuticle of my thumb. 'You know I've been trying. I've seen a million doctors.'

'We're not working, nothing is working. Your sadness is in the walls. It's impossible to be here without feeling it. I need to get on with my life.'

'But ... without me?'

She said nothing, grabbing the handle of her suitcase.

'Don't you understand? I'm sick.'

Her voice almost broke into panting. 'I kind of care about what's wrong with you, but I also really don't. I want to care more, but I just can't.'

'What can I say?'

'There's nothing. Not any more.'

Her serious, tear-stained face. She said she was going to live with her friend Rommy, an architecture student, before finding her own place. The moving van was outside. I offered to help her with her things, to pull myself together and show off some practical skills. But she only let me watch as the moving guys did all the work.

'Look how well the boxes fit in,' I said. 'They're kind of snug in there. They remind me of the time I saw Donald Judd's artwork for the first time, you know, the —'

'Shut up. Stop being such a sap.'

Before she left, I told her that I was still in love with her, but she said nothing in return, only hugging me in a limp fashion before driving away without waving back.

In our flat, with half the furniture and wall hangings and cutlery now gone, I sat alone in the filthy kitchen and then, after a long time, I lay down, my head on one of the pleated velvet cushions she hadn't wanted. On this comfortable leftover, frozen in place, I felt my despair deepen, all the way down to the bottom.

Maria was my harbour. How could I go on without her? Her face, with its mixture of wisdom and yearning, was a respite from my crippling torment and pain. She was integral not only to my life, but to the future plans for my life. I'd believed, in my bones, that the blessing of her love and companionship and our deep understanding of one another would continue until our deaths, whether they be imminent or in old age. But my love for her, which had sustained, renewed and, to a large extent, protected me, was not enough to reach across the dead white space that had grown between us, not enough to tackle and explain the nightmare of my illness.

Maybe she would always have left me. I'll never know. But it was the illness that pushed her, that took her love from me. My heart was broken now too, and wrecked among its sordid, bitter pieces, I feared that not only had the illness stripped away my sense of self, but it had taken something even greater: my ability to love.

3

Uncomfortably Numb

The battery in the hall clock died. I needed to get out of the city. Months passed, and with the promise of summer, I thought seriously about moving to Los Angeles. My friend Davika kept calling to entice me with tales of the sun and kimchi salad. But I was completely broke and, more than that, I feared my symptoms could get worse, not better. London was harsh, and stained with my heartbreak. Still, I knew its streets – or at least the ones close to my flat. Even at my worst, I could navigate them and find my way home. That sense of familiarity would vanish in America.

I watched *Chinatown*, set amid the water wars of 1930s LA, and was charmed by Jack Nicholson's swagger. It sparked something in me, and I wrote out a list of pros and cons.

In the end, the promise of friendship tipped the scale. After some grovelling at the bank, I took out a loan and booked a one-way ticket. Davika picked me up at LAX and we listened to Joanna Newsom all along the coast, windows down. The illness remained a mystery to me, but I felt a renewed sense of possibility. If London had taught me anything, it was that I could keep searching, and perhaps California would be more than a mirage – maybe even be a boon.

Davika was a hairdresser to B-list movie stars and played keyboards in a band called the Shampoo Hounds. We lived above a garage in Orange County, a neighbourhood full of sunlit porches and American flags. From the kitchen table, almost the moment I recovered from jet lag, I began to long for Maria, just as I had in London. Moving cities did little to quash my need for love and support, or my belief we should get back together. But I wanted to start a new life in LA, and I tried to spare Davika my mysterious psychodrama.

It didn't last long.

One night, gripped by the great hand, I crawled into the shower with my clothes on and sat up against the tiles, pulling my knees up to my chest. Something was different, not like my earlier episodes – I was completely numb. From my toes to the top of my skull, there was nothing, no sensations.

How utterly strange and terrifying this was.

For those of us with the use our limbs, it is one thing to

experience numbness from a temporary lack of blood flow, from sitting too long without movement or from pinched nerves. It's quite another to find yourself numb as a result of being depersonalised. The illness binds physical and emotional numbness to the point where it is all-encompassing. In the shower, I felt no tingling in my body, and no dull, pulsating aches. While there was a profound loss of feeling – when I pierced the base of my foot with a pair of nail clippers it didn't register – it is not the symptom's chief characteristic. The numbness is caused by being so dissociated from the body that any sensations feel like they are happening to somebody else.

I desperately needed to recover emotion, to be given a sharp and indisputable reminder of existence.

'We need to call the ambulance,' I said, pulling my knees in tighter.

Davika sat cross-legged outside the shower, hands restless in her lap. She had turned out all the lights and covered the digital clocks with towels. 'Do you want to go to the hospital again? You hate those lights, remember.'

'I don't think I have a choice.'

She reached for my hand, but I wouldn't take it, shrinking into the corner.

'Nathan,' she said, firmly. 'I'm going to get help.'

I listened to the door shutting behind her, feet descending on the stairs. Now she was out in the street, beginning to run, her steps fading in my ears. In a wild motion, I stood up, balancing against the tiles, and darted across the apartment in the dark, emptying the emergency pills into my hand: a mix of Valium, Zyprexa and codeine. I was breathing heavily and tripped a little on the way back to the shower. The pills spilt around the drain and I knelt over it, crying now, picking them up one by one and placing them on my tongue, swallowing without water. A couple clung to my throat and I barely coughed them up.

Paradoxically, along with the numbness came great pain, which gripped me completely. It wouldn't let up. I began to float. This pain wasn't my self fighting itself. It was the pain of my inability to fight.

One would assume that a truly all-encompassing inability to feel emotions would also include the inability to feel pain, but the paradox with feeling numb when you are depersonalised is that it causes extreme pain and suffering. We define 'pain' – from the Latin *poena*, or 'penalty', and later, the French *peine*, meaning 'suffering' – as punishment. *Penalty* makes sense. The penalty of my disease was that I had no unity of self. And no continuity of self either. We often think of numbness as a kind of radical passivity, where parts of the body shut down. But with depersonalisation, the opposite is true. The absence of emotions becomes a major source of pain, which is so great that it induces paralysis. One patient with the illness, a 24-year-old teacher who complained of persistent numbness, developed habits to affirm her existence: 'I sometimes smack my hand or pinch my leg just to feel something, and to know it's there.'

After maybe ten minutes, I can't be sure how long, two voices came up the stairs. Davika knelt on the border between the shower and the floorboards, surprisingly calm. 'Do you remember Rhonda? She's our neighbour from up the block.' Davika then explained that her friend had trained in psychotherapy.

Rhonda stepped inside the shower and slowly turned on the tap, running her hand under the water to make sure it was warm. Then, she turned the shower so that the water ran down the wall, away from me. Slowly, the space became warm with steam, and within the steam, she pushed up my trouser legs and pulled off my socks. 'Talk to us,' she whispered, 'help us understand.'

At the time, I didn't know how to describe the strange relationship between my numbness and pain. I had no idea they were symptoms of depersonalisation. What were the requirements of my pain to be considered legible beyond my own experience? How could I have known these requirements?

—

Something was happening to me in this city. The numbness was constant. It didn't seem to fluctuate, like my other symptoms. I was also having blackouts, or half-blackouts or brain shudders. When I had the energy, I walked to the pharmacy a few blocks over, chatting with one of the assistants about vitamin supplements and natural health remedies. Walking the return trip in the heat, I became acutely aware of how numb I felt. I wanted California on my eyelids, I needed it, but while I registered the feeling, I could never *really feel* it.

Nothing mattered more to me than getting better. All I wanted to talk about were my symptoms. If I could only explain them, tease them out in the right voice, I might understand them. But I limited telling Davika about the state I was in. She had heard it all before, over the phone from London, and been updated on my many hopeless visits to the doctor. Now that I was in LA, there was an unspoken agreement between us that she was not to be my nurse.

Instead, we strolled through strange neighbourhoods at dusk or drove along the freeways, turning off to take photographs of Hawaiian restaurants. Sometimes we were tempted to go through red lights, but then just sat staring up at the billboards in silence. We would drive for hours, stopping only when seduced by the neon of a gas station.

Lying in bed at night, my mind returned to all the doctors. Maybe Dr A was right when she suggested it was childhood trauma, or Dr P when he suggested bipolar; perhaps my split self was, in fact, an oscillation between mania on the one hand and low mood on the other. But I kept going back to the comments from one doctor, a thin man with a reedy voice and smooth grey moustache. He said that my symptoms were likely caused by a build-up of excess fluid in the brain, which causes intracranial pressure – what patients sometimes call 'a hard skull'. This stuck with me. His sense of certainty. My brain did, at times, feel hot and swollen.

I wanted to get a scan, but in America, because I was not a citizen, and had no insurance, embracing a new round of doctor visits was prohibitively expensive. Instead, I turned to patient testimonies online, particularly those that spoke of symptoms of numbness and pain. Unlike when I first encountered these portals, I now read with less judgement, more sadness. Many of the blog posts homed in on symptoms ('Why do I have no feeling in my head?' and 'Anybody else have a dead feeling from the chin down?'), while others took to decoding specific medical studies. I scrolled endlessly, exhausted and overwhelmed.

One post on numbness quoted Jean-Paul Sartre's *Being and Nothingness*: 'I see my hand touching objects, but do not *know* it in its act of touching them.' Sylvia Plath was there too: 'I am not solid, but hollow. I feel behind my eyes a numb, paralyzed cavern, a pit of hell, mimicking nothingness.'

———

Before the concert, Davika kept looking at her watch. Her keyboard and amp were crammed into the van, set list in her pocket. At the prospect of a night out, I rode a wave of happiness. But Davika drove so fast on the freeway, forgetting to indicate when changing lanes, that I held my breath, jaw stiff. It was a strange gig. We entered through an old storefront to a concrete back lot. A goth band was playing to about forty people, the crowd a smattering of black woollen hats and eyeliner. I felt out of place in my fresh trousers. The Shampoo Hounds were halfway into their set, the crowd shouting 'Shampoo! Shampoo!' when I saw Rhonda. It was the first time since the night in the shower. After the concert, she invited the band, and me, back to her house.

'I have a pool,' she said, shaking her keys lightly in her palm.

She saw a look of uncertainty on my face and glanced quickly aside.

The pool was surrounded by lights and little palms. A fresh, cold smell of chlorine filled the air. The band jumped in and out of the water in their underwear, stopping to do cocaine and eat raspberry yoghurt out of one big tub. Wet feet slapped the tiles. I envied their abandon as they climbed onto one another's backs and threw beer cans, singing lines from old country songs.

Shadows moved. I froze.

Davika tried to coax me into the water, her hand waving me in.

Looking down at the tiles, I mumbled, 'Not right now.'

Never again.

My experience at the poolside was happening to somebody else. Wait. It wasn't like that. My body was firmly in place, but I was separated from its sensations. I was numb. This caused a deep pain, which began in my stomach and spread out beyond the border of my skin, becoming a capsule of pain. My body grew larger, taking up more space. A part of me was reaching out for something, beyond the capsule, which made those around me – Davika, Rhonda, the band – grow smaller.

Feeling numb and in pain came on when I caught sight of the water, which triggered a memory of my onset. Although I was in a different city, some of the conditions were the same. It was late and dark; spontaneous. The water promised glee and delight but was now a site of terror.

'Where are you going?' shouted Davika.

I wasn't aware of stepping slowly backwards. 'Nowhere.'

Although the water was shallow and well lit, I didn't want to be one of the drowning soldiers. I didn't want to gasp for air, longing for home. If I touched the surface of the pool, even for a second, the waves would pull me under, and I would be lost among bodies and the battleship's debris. Reassurance was tough. My inner voice was against me. Still, I tried. I was not a man in uniform, I told myself, not a person from the textbooks. Instead, I was surrounded by friends in a peaceful suburban backyard.

I had no language for this pain. But I didn't doubt it, which was strange, because I was uncertain of so much else. When we think of pain in the body emanating from a particular place, it becomes easier to assess. For my stomach pain, a doctor might order stool samples or conduct an endoscopy. For my chest pain, there might be an x-ray or heart monitor. To date, though, the results of such tests had yielded little. This, I felt, was a denial of my testimony. When a doctor couldn't locate the trouble, then, ergo, I was not in pain. As for many depersonalisation sufferers, the gap between my own narrative and the clinic's scepticism left me alone and afraid.

For psychologist Theodore Barber, pain has two components: sensory and affective. Pain might be an aching, burning, prickling sensation, but it also includes a reaction pattern. This is our concern about the pain. Barber calls it *the pain affect*. Here's the interesting thing: for those with depersonalisation, the components get caught in a loop. The dog, sensation, chases its tail, the affective response to pain. But because the source of pain in the body is difficult to locate, the sensory signals try again, to no avail. The reaction, now, is one of distress and a further, frantic search for the source.

———

For all its famous sprawl, LA felt like a cul-de-sac. Touching down in California, I naively hoped for invitations to the Chateau Marmont or Musso & Frank's. Some unexpected event to turn the tide. But my days involved little more than walking to the pharmacy for Advil and Excedrin. Apart from Davika, who worked long hours, I rarely saw anyone. Even when I couldn't leave the house, I tried not to slump on the lounge. Being numb, it was important to keep active.

I thought often of Maria. The memory of our earliest days wouldn't leave me: the exquisite pleasure that came from her smile, the way she swept along the pavement in her black dress, the way her hand hovered delicately over a D minor chord on the piano, the tender way she spoke about her mother, the studious way she would take a pad of drawing paper out on the grass and try to capture the joy of picnickers in charcoal, the careful way she sipped a frosted glass of cranberry juice, and the curl of her vowels when she said 'avenue' and 'eardrum'. I was in awe of what our love had been. It promised value. And refuge. I was convinced that reclaiming it could be my lifeline.

What I didn't know was that the partners of depersonalised patients often have trouble dealing with how the illness changes relationships. For the sufferer, it is hard to articulate their symptoms, and for the partner it can be near impossible to comprehend, let alone offer the necessary support.

Kevin Burdette, a 42-year-old man whose wife, Constance, was diagnosed with depersonalisation, said his marriage fell apart when his wife's symptoms became all-consuming. 'I couldn't cope. Everything we'd built for our life seemed to go away when she got sick. She couldn't go outside because she said everything outside wasn't real. All the roads didn't make sense to her any more. Being around her every day took a serious toll on my own health, and I was being pulled into her lack of reality. I felt I had no choice but to leave. When we signed the divorce papers, I was heartbroken because she said she couldn't feel anything. She had no emotions.'

Another partner I spoke to, a 22-year-old woman who worked as a trainee accountant, told me that right after she got engaged to her boyfriend he had an onset of depersonalisation. 'I knew he was going to be in for the long haul with this thing and so I had to decide if I would stay or not. It might sound harsh but I ended up saying "Fuck it" and moved on. I couldn't live with him any more, not when he was like that. Every night at dinner he said he wasn't inside his body any more. Tell me somebody who can live with a guy who says shit like that.'

One morning I woke late to the burr of traffic and decided to call Maria. She was at a bus stop in East London. Her phone kept breaking up.

'What are you talking about?' she said, after my opening monologue.

'It has to do with ... with ... that first time we kissed on the lawn.'

She softened, slowing her words like a teacher does with a delinquent. 'I'm sorry. I don't want to be mean to you.'

'It's my health.'

'But it's hard to take your illness seriously. I still don't understand what's wrong. How can you be totally numb? Every time you talk about it I'm more confused.'

The more I pleaded for help and recognition the more it seemed to falter. She could never understand what was happening to me and I was foolish to court her sympathy. I needed someone to sift through the possibilities, a partner to help with my quest. But she never signed up for that.

'I wish I knew what was wrong,' I said, a sob rising in my throat. 'But we can find each other again, and get our love back.'

Her pause, which must have lasted only a few seconds, was three hours long. Finally she said, 'I don't want that.'

Hurt flooded my face. 'You can't really mean —'

'I do,' she said, a hint of emotion creeping in.

'If you don't love me, it doesn't matter. I can find the love for the both of —'

'Stop it. If you're honest with yourself, calling me is selfish. It's not about us, it's about you being sick.' Her bus pulled into the stop, brakes creaking, doors opening with a single loud *pah*. 'And our relationship – what we were – won't fix that.'

———

My need for distraction after this defeat was intense. But I didn't regret contacting Maria again. The spectre of our early love had grown too powerful. Facing it was important. Still, being so humbled made me even more antisocial. I sat at my desk trying to read research papers for my thesis. On good days, I would write, which animated me. Writing helped make sense of my environment, improving my spatial awareness. I think this rebalancing was a result of working through what I saw in the world – shape, language, colour – and marking my place within it. It grounded me physically: 'I am sitting at this desk, writing.'

More often, though, my perception was foggy. I couldn't concentrate on the page for more than ten minutes without my eyelids drooping with fatigue. One afternoon I was jolted out of my stupor by a woman talking loudly in the street. She was back from a holiday and spoke about the cool orange groves by the sea in Italy and how the trees were still and golden in the summer heat. I thought of Maria. If we could only share such an experience, walk together on a sparkling trail, then maybe, just maybe, her love for me would return.

It was clear. I couldn't let go. I had no reason to believe Maria would ever love me again, but my mind persisted in longing for her. French novelist Stendhal described the involuntary nature of this longing: 'Love is like a fever which comes and goes quite independently of the will.' Unrequited love is even worse: 'If in the midst of pleasure we are wrenched away from it, suffering will result.' My love for Maria was hope, of which I was in desperate need. Even though she was now gone, to move on from her would mean abandoning the sense of stability she once provided. I couldn't afford that.

Davika suggested I try something new: Las Vegas. Her band was playing a few dates in a club off the strip. Reluctantly, I joined her in the van. My pockets were full of blister packs that made popping noises at sharp turns. I sipped Diet Pepsi and counted cars. On the outskirts of LA, the city began to fall away, leaving cracked parking lots and t-shirt vendors behind for the expanse of the desert. We passed a sandy mountain range and plains of shrubs. Lanes opened up, out and out. This time, car travel at high speed was soothing. The engine caught up to my brain and cooled my thoughts. My body sank lightly into the seat as a song about an old pair of boots came on the radio. Waves of melody poured over me.

I wanted to remain inside this calm and shut my eyes.

When you are numb as a result of depersonalisation, reality is contingent. You are always waiting to *feel* reality, for a hard, implacable thing to announce itself, for a gear shift or big brown rock to look and feel how you expect it to. With this sense of reality will also come – you hope – the knowledge that the world has a place for you. The thought is: if reality is no longer contingent, if it is *really real*, then I, too, am real because I am inside this reality. In a strange way, you wait for reality to feel you back.

Living in this limbo state causes fear. You are poised for change but it never comes. One depersonalisation patient, a 22-year-old postman, was with his friends when it suddenly struck him they were ghosts. He was caught between two worlds: the real and the unreal. He couldn't break out. The fear of being in this state was all-consuming, to the point of his hospitalisation.

Another patient, a 27-year-old Brazilian woman, was consumed with fear when she couldn't feel her body. She described it as being 'somewhere else and hollow, with nothing but the skin, and it seemed to be someone else's body'. To reduce her fear of being unreal, she wore bracelets to mark the boundaries of her limbs.

When I was inside the car, my dread was easier to bear. I was still numb, but the rumble of hard tyres over the bitumen diluted my fear of being trapped in that state forever.

At sunset, the dirt shimmered. We stopped in a border town and decided to stay the night. Our hotel doubled as a casino. It was a worn brick building trying its luck with a few slot machines in the front room. The place was empty. A friendly couple met us at the front desk, giving us a copy of *The Plan of Salvation* with our room keys.

'Mormons,' said Davika, as we unpacked our bags. 'They own a lot of casinos here.'

I didn't see the pool until morning. As I pulled back the curtains, my fear returned in a great rush, bubbling up into my throat.

I looked away. I looked back.

'No soldiers,' I said, gasping, my breath visible on the window.

A diving board hovered over one end. Pale, blue and cracked. Covered in early mist, it cut through the morning, breaking up the sun, a dividing line between the world and the water. I felt myself in two parts. One part of myself was outside the water. The other – my confined self, the piece broken away from me – was somewhere in the space of the pool. My numbness embedded itself deeper, burrowing south into another layer. What was this layer?

Pain.

Why did the mere sight of water now deepen my feeling of not having a self? I was becoming more sensitised. Water was a key element of my onset, and being exposed to it only reinforced the severity of my symptoms. As my numbness grew, so did my pain.

Studies suggest that patients experiencing depersonalisation with persistent numbness often exhibit pain asymbolia, also called pain dissociation. In such cases, the patient will acknowledge the sensation of pain but report that it doesn't belong to them. Several researchers, including Irene Tracey at Oxford University and Vania Apkarian at Northwestern University, have proposed that this type of pain can be understood by looking at discrete signatures of brain activity. These are identified using advanced neuroimaging techniques and help show how emotional and cognitive factors shape pain perception.

In her lab at Oxford, Tracey uses the 3-Tesla MRI scanner to show the significant differences between acute pain – like that caused by sunburn or bruising – and chronic pain, which persists beyond the typical healing period. When pain becomes chronic, the brain responds in fundamentally different ways. As Tracey describes it, chronic pain is 'something new, with a life of its own, its own biology, and its own mechanisms, most of which we really don't understand at all'.

What we do know is that for depersonalised patients there is often a profound reduction in the physiological response to pain. This is due to lower skin conductance in response to unpleasant stimuli. Normally when we experience something emotional, say, a near-miss car accident or being chased by a pit bull, the rush of adrenaline triggers the sweat glands, making our skin more conductive to electricity. But science shows that for those with depersonalisation, the brain's nociceptive, or pain, signals are blunted. And sometimes absent altogether. This creates a paradoxical state where the patient feels both numbness and pain simultaneously.

———

Back from Las Vegas, I stayed in bed and read at all hours. When I began to nod off, I slapped myself lightly and pressed on. The hope was to find some character, idea or metaphor that might point the way, even if only for a day or two. Davika's bookshelves were full of the European miserabilists: Camus, Kafka, Cioran, Duras. I wanted none of these sad books. I tried Jane Austen's *Emma*, which I always thought would be sunny, but it didn't take. Instead, I tackled a lively little paperback about the migratory habits of Scandinavian birds, which was sprinkled with wonderful Latin names and drawings. In the middle of the book, where the spine was coming apart, was a passage about the beauty of a Norwegian snowfall and how one bird called the willow grouse liked to flit from log to log. I wrote the bird's name in the margin and thought of this tiny free bird.

Without much of an appetite, I cooked soup in a dented pot and sucked lozenges that tasted like flowers. Light came and went from the blinds.

One friend sent me a postcard and signed off with the recommendation: 'Try Richard Yates.' When I mentioned this to Davika, she laughed and said his books were sadder than all of the miserabilists. 'But he does have an LA novel.' *Disturbing the Peace* follows an alcoholic salesman called John Wilder, who has a history of mental illness and moves to Hollywood in the hope of becoming a movie producer. Things go badly. After holing up in a motel off Sunset Boulevard, he mixes a cocktail of booze and drugs, becoming a zombie: 'He felt nothing at all, and heard nothing, and saw nothing. It came as a bewildering surprise to find he was still breathing.'

When I came to these lines I read them aloud to Davika. I needed to sound a warning: if I start to slip like Mr Wilder, be sure to tell me. Yates's novel stayed with me for weeks. I kept returning to scenes where Wilder was numb and lost to himself. The portrait of mental illness in LA was a strange, unsettling mirror. Would I end up drinking gin and tonic on a patio while the sun set over the Pacific? Or would I get into a fight with waiters at an Italian restaurant on La Cienega Boulevard and end up in the streets telling the world I killed Kennedy?

Davika snatched the book from my hands and hurled it out the window. 'It's only a novel! You are not Mr Wilder!'

I lay in bed for so long that a groove formed in the mattress. Shadows lengthened and darkened on the ceiling. I ate spaghetti on paper plates with hard crusts of bread, crumbs lodging in my body hair. One evening, when I got up to sit on the balcony, there was a sudden downpour. Water flowed out of the drains and rushed along the gutters. Across the street, a small bus pulled up and a group of scouts got out. Before the scoutmaster could properly corral them, the boys took off down the pavement in quick, clipped steps. They wore pale green raincoats and binoculars that bounced around on their boyish chests. Amid the raindrops, shouting and name-calling and scuffed knees. The boys seemed oblivious to the complex world of other people, the houses they passed that were filled with the sad air of microwave dinners, the office workers and hairdressers with impossible headaches who'd just minutes before retreated inside to hug a bottle of Maker's Mark.

I held on to the railing. It was cold and wet. I began to cry uncontrollably.

'Hey Tom! John! Brian! Wait just a —'

But the boys were already gone.

The bus was gone, the joy of their coats in the rain was gone. I cried and cried. My body shook. I mourned for the boy I once was, the boy seated between all the other boys on the back seat telling jokes about big dicks and monster whales and not thinking about the troubles of tomorrow because tomorrow didn't exist. It was only here, in this moment at the back of the bus, with all of us laughing in the warmth of our living bodies ...

I stepped off the balcony, slow on the stairs, and walked along the brick path into the garden. The smell of the cold grass rushed at my face. I lay down among the ferns and put my face into the soil.

'It's all the same life,' I said over and over, trying to believe it.

I hungered for a continuity of self, confirmation that the boy I'd been was not lost. Did my childhood live within the body now curled between the leaves? Or was it closed off from me forever?

'One life ...'

A pair of black boots entered the garden, splashing the puddles.

'I need you to cut my hair.'

Davika was standing over me with a towel.

'What?'

She used the towel to shield her head. 'You heard me.'

'But you're the hairdresser.'

'You need to get up.' She smiled and took my hand, lifted me onto my feet.

Raindrops ran down my face, dripping off my nose.

Inside, Davika sat on a plastic chair in the shower. I cut her fringe. Strands of hair built up around the drain. With each snip of the scissors, trying to keep my hands steady, I listened to the cool patter of her voice as she spoke about a new song she was working on, the new keyboard she wanted to buy, her hopes for touring and producing and one day maybe even moving to a farm in Ohio where she could build a recording studio and raise chickens.

Tears streamed down my cheeks. Her hair fell away.

For months she'd been caring for me, despite herself. The self-absorption that accompanied my illness was a serious tax, and yet her friendship persisted beyond all reasonable limits. She always listened, always asked the right questions. Her endurance of my altered state was now teaching me how to endure. Davika's greatest gift was accepting where I was, the empty space between my two selves. Her friendship, her love, let me speak from between the pieces.

4

The Invisible Baby

My mother told me the story of being pregnant with her first child – me. She was in Sydney, and the video chat kept breaking up. It was my birthday and every year she liked to tell me the same joyous tale of feeling my body inside her. I pressed on the walls of her uterus, she said, softening it, expanding it, swimming at all hours – freestyle, breaststroke, even butterfly. I kicked and splashed and took quick, sharp breaths. She said she ate nothing but tinned peaches because when she cracked the first can I rolled around, asking for more. She said I liked the tin's sharp, metallic pop.

We laughed a lot, she said, laughed and laughed. We went to the park and watched the pigeons. How noisy they were, always gossiping. I grew a little bit. We shopped for prams and decided on one with colourful dots and moons. I grew a little more. We bought too many Christmas decorations and covered the tree with so much bling that my father said we'd overdosed on Christmas. 'No more Bing Crosby!' We kissed his cranky head and he danced with us.

I grew hair and fingernails.

Sick of peaches – finally – we bought a steaming tub of Chinese takeaway and stood up against the garden shed, hot sauce on our tongues. I wouldn't stop growing.

'You were having so much fun in there,' my mother said, pointing at her stomach offscreen, her voice high in my computer speakers.

In the third trimester, we spent a week at a holiday camp by the beach. My mother wore a pale orange bikini, her big belly shining in the sun as she walked in the shallows. We swam in the mornings and the late afternoons. Ocean water got into her gums. At night, the summer heat bore down on our tent. When my mother got up to pee, mosquitoes swarmed her ankles. But there was no swatting them away. We were too big now, couldn't bend down.

The computer screen grew choppy, then froze. I could still hear her voice.

'That's not how it was for me,' I said.

'You were just a little foetus, a baby.'

'I was trapped. I couldn't get out.'

'You were happy inside me.'

The sudden urge to vomit. 'It's too disturbing. We need to stop.'

I couldn't shake the mental picture of being in my mother's womb. I was enclosed, helpless, held as if inside a tomb. But it wasn't a tomb, it was a place of life. This picture of myself, before birth, haunted me. It mirrored the part of my self in confinement. The 'me' that had been confined before birth was confined again. Sometimes, the light was different in the picture, where I could see my tiny body, and other times I was only a dark outline. I desperately wanted to change this image and break free. But the more I tried to replace the picture with others – being at the beach or in open fields – the more it cemented itself, digging deeper into my consciousness.

I wrestled with the picture, trying to tame it, dampen its hold on me.

In the middle of the night, I woke up and the picture was right in front of me, so tangible I could have touched it, reached into the dark and stroked my own foetus. I spoke to the picture, pleading with it to let me out of the womb.

Soon I entered a new stage of horror: multiple pictures. They piled up quickly. I saw myself again and again. Pale, grey, blurry. Muted, tangled, grainy. The carousel wouldn't stop. This baby, that baby, again and again, pictures slapped me, wet pictures, straight from the womb. Slap, slap, slap.

Please stop. I need to rest. Let me lie down. Just for a minute. Slap, slap, slap. The carousel turned. Babies twisting, wriggling, trying to escape, squirming in waves of fluid. *Mother, I —* The carousel sped up, light breaking the projector, each new baby passing through my skull, dropping into the dark. *But mother —* Forty babies, fifty, sixty. How many? Hundreds pierced my mind, making me stumble, eyes blinking. Okay. Is it slowing now, the endless carousel? No. Stop. Greater speed. Greater still. *But doctor – I took the pills – I did everything —* Is that baby dead? What about that one? Stop. I don't want to see this. Let me live far from this prison. Maybe music will work, slow the pictures, subdue them, loud classical music. *DA-NA-NA-NAH.* It has to work. It has to.

It's not working.

Babies in the current, thousands of them, racing into my mind with the force of an army.

A short walk became a marathon. The great hand treated me like a puppet, pressing me into the pavement. My legs turned to stone. Each new step was a herculean effort. I concentrated on my shoes, willing them to help me.

'I need to buy milk and oil,' I said, repeating my task aloud.

Houses all around me: gutters and drains. They looked like a Cubist painting, broken up. I stumbled and leaned on a pole. All the palm trees and Hondas in the driveways were fuzzy. The street signs were even stranger. NO PARKING and KEEP OUT collided with the baby pictures. One baby crashed into BEWARE OF DOG while another slammed into NO JUNK MAIL. My mind couldn't process the real world and the pictures together. My vision was a collage. But it wasn't static. The collage shifted constantly, skittish and jumpy. Each new baby obstructed my view, erasing key elements of the world I needed to anchor reality.

When I finally got back to the house, I fainted.

When I came to, I drank some milk.

The air smelt of moist stones, moss and water.

I fainted again.

———

Depersonalisation often makes a person prone to philosophical thinking, posing tortured questions about existence and the unitary self. Am I real? How is it possible to know I am real when my stable sense of self is gone? If I am *not* real, unable to see my face in the mirror as my own, how can I be sure that the world exists? Was theologian John Henry Newman right when he asked: 'If we cannot see ourselves as "I", how can we possibly see the world of creation?'

For family and friends, these questions quickly become irritating and exhausting. The depersonalisation patient speaks on a loop and, despite assurances, their thoughts are repeated in an attempt to control a serious decline in mental health. Nothing seems to calm the need for absolute confirmation of reality. But how do we provide this? Some resort to ridicule, reducing the person to a caricature of teen angst. This does great harm to relationships. Because the disease is not widely known, it's easy to dismiss it as hypochondria or malingering. For me, and others who are depersonalised, questions about existence are an attempt to understand our symptoms, essential to comprehending what is happening to us. Our self-absorption is the result of having no self.

Where am I? Where did I come from before birth? Where will I go after death?

Growing up, I thought these things were settled, that certain long-standing questions that have occupied us down the ages would remain unanswered. Until the onset of my illness, I'd accepted my lack of answers and, like most of us, moved on. Necessity demanded it. But now these questions came at me with the force of a jet plane.

I thought deeply about those who kill themselves. Where are they now? If I am already dead, living outside my shell of a body, how is my existence any different? Are we alive – do we share this world – or is this sense we have of life a dream that never happened?

In his book *The Theory of Moral Sentiments*, economist and philosopher Adam Smith suggested that these strange

questions are perfectly understandable when we are con-
fronted with mortality. To manage the fear of death, we use
our imagination to sympathise with the dead. This makes us
their companions. We think about what they have lost and
it terrifies us: 'It is miserable, we think, to be deprived of the
light of the sun; to be shut out from life and conversation; to
be laid in the cold grave, a prey to corruption and the reptiles
of the earth; to be no more thought of in this world, but to
be obliterated.'

Sympathy is how we develop fellow feeling with others.
In life, we share feelings of grief and fear to cope with
the challenges of the mortal hour. But we cannot console the
dead. They do not know what we feel, nor do they care.
Instead, our sympathy for the non-living triggers a troubling
feedback loop as we project our lives onto those who can
offer nothing back. We take on their misery and commune
with the afterlife.

In someone who is depersonalised, sympathy for the dead
is particularly acute. Hardly a day passes without them con-
sidering the question of existence. The way this presents in
their mind is different from their high-speed thinking in other
episodes. Everything is slow and loud. Nothing slips by. Each
new thought ('Are the dead whole again?' 'Is the self finally
at peace?' 'What is it like to reach the end of consciousness?')
is seen clearly, as if spelled out on a giant, flapping banner.

The mind sinks into these thoughts, having little choice but to contemplate them.

I thought constantly about the meaning of silence. Only the dead know it. In life, silence is never absolute. When a parent tells their child to be silent, it is not because they believe it is possible, only that they wish for less noise. When the child is asleep in the cot, there is still the sound of them breathing and snoring, and the babble induced by dreams. Although we try our best to be silent, it only acts as a container for sound. Attempts to pray or meditate are met with traffic in the distance, rain on the roof, the rustle of clothing. Soundproof a room only to hear the buzz of cables and lights. Even in solitary confinement, a prisoner must hear their own sighs.

Being raised in the Christian tradition, I was taught that silence is important precisely because it is impossible. Only God can be truly silent. We, the living, might aspire to silence, but only God can grant it – in death. In my dark, sluggish thinking, I thought of growing up in the presence of the Bible, and how at the dinner table my parents would remind me that the dead surround us. They are always present. Why? Because the dead belong to God, and God is always present.

In my struggle with the illness, I didn't want to have sympathy for the dead. I wanted to be cured. To laugh and laugh and laugh. Growing up I had a neighbour, Mrs Pine, who used to say that forcing yourself to laugh increased the chance of it happening naturally. Her idea was that performance will become a reality. I tried this. But I was too sick to bridge the gap. My throat produced the sound, but it was hollow in the air.

I couldn't recognise my own voice.

———

The driveway was lined with hedges and statues. I hadn't been to a house party in years, and I wanted to prove to myself, and Davika, that I could be social. When we moved inside, there were people dancing barefoot and drinking beer among tall plants. The smell of pot pervaded the halls. I was wearing a vintage Malibu t-shirt and a new pair of Chuck Taylor sneakers with signature stripes. We wandered between thin girls with inky skulls on their necks, and past a buffet where hipsters took tiny bites out of beet burgers while the Gossip song 'Heavy Cross' played from hidden speakers. For a brief moment, my legs were loose and free. But then something in the air changed. I became paranoid that people were looking at me, whispering about me, saying that my body was strange and misshapen, that there were two of me staring at them. I ran out of the main room and fled upstairs, swallowing some pills when I reached the landing.

In an empty bedroom, I found a walk-in closet and came face to face with a wall of baby pictures. There must have been fifty – colour, black and white – in all different sizes. It was like falling into a cage of spiders. The babies were trapped in their frames. So still. At first. Then they began to move, wriggling limbs and legs, heads nodding and turning.

I was pulled inside one of the frames. It was hard, immovable.

Nothing about this was normal. I wasn't supposed to be back in the womb or in a picture frame. This was a party. There should be ice in my drink. What is the clock doing? I can't see the time from in here. It's never been this late. *I told you I can't see.* The red digits are blinking, numbers and hours changing. The babies are whispering. *But doctor —* They are saying I will never get out. *But doctor, I thought —* There is no map to navigate the coils of the womb. Forget your freedom. Give in to these walls.

I ran onto the balcony and threw up, just missing a group of dancers. Someone shouted at me from below. When I turned around, the party's host was in my face. He told me to get the fuck out of his mother's room. I apologised and fled, taking the stairs two at a time, running into Davika with vomit on my chin.

The return of the baby carousel was even worse this time. The slap, slap, slap was faster and the pictures more vivid. But my response was different. Instead of recoiling at the pictures, I thought of ways to confront them. My quest was to tame the carousel, bring it to a halt. I felt that if I could see myself inside my mother's womb, I would know I was real. In establishing the reality of me, I could reclaim my unitary self. I could return to one, true body. But my mother assured me there was no ultrasound. They didn't give you pictures to take home, she said. Not back then.

I wasn't convinced.

One morning, in my distress, I called the hospital where I was born. A nurse on the ward was polite and helpful. She asked for the date of birth, saying it shouldn't be a problem. They kept images on file. When I said '1980', the line went quiet. She asked me to repeat the date.

'I'm sorry, sir. Those records don't exist any more. We only keep pictures for three months. I don't think there was —'

I sharpened a pencil and drew myself. If there was no picture of me, I would draw my own, the way it was inside. I drew a circle, a box, another circle. I used so much of my eraser that white shavings covered my palm. The notebook filled up. I drew my face, arms, limbs. I drew my feet, the umbilical cord. I drew my hands, which never looked right. But I kept trying. I desperately needed to feel okay with the concrete image of myself in the womb. Only then could I help the infant I was break free.

The notebook wasn't enough. I needed to see evidence of my birth, that I'd made it into the world. This led me to watch birthing videos. Many were overly sanitised and used for educational purposes. What I needed was raw and real. I found one on YouTube called 'Window Water Baby Moving', a video the artist Stan Brakhage took of his wife Jane giving birth. The footage was from the 1950s, with a pink-fleshy cast. Jane panted and convulsed. In a close-up of the birth canal, the baby's head edged out and out. I couldn't look away. The umbilical cord was finally cut and the tiny body began to wail. I put my hand on the screen and traced the baby's outline.

When a person becomes distraught by the experience of having no self, it probably shouldn't surprise us that they commonly fixate on birth. It works in tandem with suicide ideation. When given a brief respite from thinking about death, the mind turns to an obsession with birth, and how the self – now lost – first came to be. We rarely associate mourning with birth. We mourn those who have died. But for the depersonalised, who *feel* like they have died, there is a mourning for birth too.

One patient, a 42-year-old mother, found herself reduced to a foetus-like state. She was always hungry. The problem was that despite adequate food and drink, she never felt the fullness in her stomach. It was 'as if the content were not going in'. She became fixated on life's earliest, primal need:

food from her pregnant mother. Another patient couldn't feel the sensation of food and drink either. Nutrients from outside the womb suddenly ceased to matter. The only 'real' food was delivered before birth. The interesting thing is that these patients had no desire to return to the womb. They did not want to be trapped, did not want to be born again. They wanted to die, to end the need for food once and for all.

What intrigues me is how birth relates to the self. When we are born, our physical body enters the world. Our brain enters too. According to philosopher Martin Heidegger, the self is defined by its ability to interrogate itself. The self can wonder at its being. But a newborn's cognitive capacities are not yet sophisticated enough to do this, which means the self is born sometime after birth.

The consensus is that it occurs in early childhood. Some psychologists say age two, others about four or five. In this phase, we develop a sense of self by recognising ourselves in mirrors and photos. We understand ourselves as separate from our mother and know our thoughts and feelings as our own.

The question arises: what happens to the self in the gap between birth and early childhood? Is it lost, or simply waiting? Before we see the baby in the mirror, who is that baby? It's hard to believe more people are not fascinated by this mysterious pocket of time, but it can be very distressing for those with depersonalisation. The idea of seeing the world and breathing its air without having a self is unbearable. More frightening is to imagine a child in this state – a helpless creature bereft.

———

LA is not a religious place. Hollywood draws everything into its vortex with such power that there's never much oxygen for divinity. I longed for spiritual connection, somewhere my loneliness would be received without shame or judgement. Out under the palms of Sunset or Franklin, I'd imagine myself back in England, climbing the steps of the Brompton Oratory to sit quietly in the pews. I listened for the creak of the door behind the altar and the sounds of priests lighting candles in the sacristy.

Traffic roared, then slowed.

I started reading about sightings of the Virgin Mary. She appeared to a Belgian woman in 1859 and said, 'Go and fear nothing, I will help you.' Two decades later she appeared on a church wall in the Irish village of Knock, and for an hour, glowed in silence, surrounded by angels. In the twentieth century she appeared to children in Portugal, teenagers in Brazil and a Dutch secretary named Ida Peerdeman, to whom she said, 'Woman, behold your son.'

The idea of a supernatural mother was deeply appealing. It offered an escape from the wreck of my thoughts. The Virgin was the opposite of the great hand. Every instance I read of her appearances provided comfort and aid. She was a hand infused not with darkness, but goodness and light. I wanted her to guide me back to my self, for her to say, 'Be at peace,' as she had to the parishioners of the Irish church.

Before the onset of my illness, I would have sniggered at tales of the Virgin appearing in forests and churches. But my symptoms made me think it was possible. I was living in some kind of purgatory, which implied there must be a space – a realm – where the Virgin existed too. When reality is upended, it becomes possible to entertain all kinds of mystical possibilities. I was more open to the supernatural than ever.

'When my friend died in high school and I didn't want to talk to anyone, I read a book by Saint Teresa at lunch.' Davika stood tall against the kitchen cabinet. She finished her glass of beer then lifted her head, placing fingertips at her temples. 'It was a weird old book, kind of like her auto-biography. The title was something like The Eternal Castle, or maybe The Internal Castle. She wrote in one chapter about seeing the Virgin all dressed in white. Anyway, if I can remember it right, she thinks that the castle is the self, or the soul, and outside the castle is all the dirt of society. If you don't want the self to get dirty you have to keep it safe.' She spoke with enviable lightness and care. 'When you talk about your symptoms and that you're split in two and don't know yourself, it makes sense the way she wrote about everything, that we end up losing ourselves and have to try to find it again.' She opened the fridge and pulled out a jar of green olives and another beer. 'People still think they see Mary all the time. There's a place up north, way out in the desert.'

When I researched the site, I saw that she was right. Since 1990, the Virgin had appeared to many people at a rock in the Mojave Desert. Families with sick children and those seeking absolution gathered to wait for a sign. On a sun-drenched afternoon, I plucked up the confidence to drive. This wasn't easy. I hesitated, and pulled over constantly to rest. In the end, I spent hours navigating unmarked roads before I found the spot. A few people were taking photographs. Some were carrying prints. One person told me the Virgin revealed herself in patterns of light; another had heard her voice on the wind.

Sunlight moved over the rock, throwing off reflections and shadows. It cast a strange spell. I couldn't look away. The yellowish, sandy texture hid something within. It was pitted with smooth holes and grooves, worn away by the seasons, and reminded me of da Vinci's painting *Virgin of the Rocks*, which hangs in London's National Gallery – the Virgin is perched at the base of a craggy monolith, hand outstretched.

I stood where so many of the hopeless and lost had been before me. The knowledge that I was in a space of collective longing, that this spot, *right here*, was a place of hope, blunted any cynicism I might have had. The light changed, and I begged the Virgin to appear. I needed to be healed, made whole. I would do anything.

'Our Lady, please, on this rock ...'

When we think about mental illness and religion, the association is often of a person going mad. A full-blown psychosis can induce hallucinations: Jesus is coming; Satan has arrived; angels are singing. For the depersonalised, there are no such hallucinations. The voices are internal, not external. Here's the paradox: people with depersonalisation know that their feelings of detachment and lost self are *not* real, whereas many with a psychotic disorder believe their feelings to be reality. While depersonalisation shares some symptoms with schizophrenia and bipolar disorder (particularly the sense of the body being invaded and vacated), it doesn't rob the person of sanity. The patient is always conscious of their unreality.

According to Dr Krast, a psychiatrist who specialises in treating depersonalisation, making the distinction between internal and external voices is integral for reaching a correct diagnosis. Krast tells the story of Evan, a 29-year-old patient with a history of troubling internal voices. 'Evan is not psychotic. He has intact "reality testing" about his depersonalisation: he knows ... that his unusual perceptions are just subjective experiences that are not "real" other than for his internal world. A person with psychosis would not only feel as if he was leaving his body but would believe that this is in effect happening.'

In longing for the Virgin to appear, I imagined her voice. But I did not believe that I *heard* her voice. I wanted salvation, to be given a heavenly sign, but I never felt one was there.

Driving out of the desert, I replayed my encounter with the rock, circling it in my mind. As I turned back for LA, my vision grew blurry. I pulled over in a picnic area. A group of women were preparing lunch, laying out a tablecloth with paper plates and napkins. They had just arrived, and it became clear some were strangers meeting for the first time. Soft music played from a radio. Around a bench, they opened crackers and jams and strips of turkey meat, laughing and shaking hands. One woman picked her baby up out of the pram, and said, 'This is my son.'

———

Mothers are born every day. In childbirth, a mother, too, arrives. Every minute that passes, a woman, somewhere, has a child placed in her arms. The bright hospital lights. The sight of blood on a white towel. She can't stop blinking. In the street, the cars and the trees – nothing looks the same. Nothing sounds the same either. There is now another voice in the crowd. One that cries out for sustenance and direction.

I began to mistake faces in the supermarket for my mother. Walking down by the long bank of freezers, with their tall foggy doors, I saw my mother buying milk, crossing off a shopping list with a tiny pencil. She looked so young, her long, thick hair catching her shoulders. But it wasn't her. Down another aisle, I saw my pregnant mother. I was sure of it. But how could it be? She wore a long, red coat, and was pushing a trolley. *Wait* — Did she really just pop up here in southern California holding that plastic bag of corn?

She appeared again, so old, her scalp visible under her thin hair. Toothpaste. There were too many options. But she needed to choose. My mother held several in her hands, squinting, before dropping them all. A teenage employee helped her pick them up and for a second, she glanced up at me, embarrassed. I smiled at her.

Walking home, I was thinking about the different faces of my mother when a huge semi-trailer raced by and sprayed mud all over me. The brown sludge covered my hands, dripping from my fingers. I wiped them on the glass of a bus shelter. But I couldn't get them dry. The mud was too thick. I ran across the road to a gas station bathroom and held them under the hot blast of the dryer.

Sliding down the wall, I closed my eyes. The air was stale and smelt of feet. Sirens wailed outside. I counted to ten, twenty, thirty. 'It's daytime,' I said, my voice an echo in the tiny space, a reminder that I was far from the Hampstead pond.

Back at the house, I continued drying my hands. Somehow, they were still wet: a drop of water on my palm, a speck of mud on my wrist, a damp streak between my thumb and forefinger. I dried them so hard that my skin flaked off. I started to bleed. Only then, at the sight of blood, did I stop.

It was an everyday event: a truck spraying mud. But it signalled a line had been crossed, that LA was not the sanctuary I'd hoped it would be, that its lights were only a mirage, that wherever I tried to run I could never escape my illness. I thought of Jonah. He, too, tried to run. Ignoring God's word, he fled the city and was swallowed by the whale. Only his prayers saved him from drowning.

Davika stood against the doorframe, sipping a milkshake. 'What am I going to do if you leave?'

I sat on my hands. 'Have a break from me.'

She laughed softly at this remark, then took out her straw and sucked the base of it. 'I don't want you to go.'

'I think I might need to do more tests.'

She shook her head. 'There's no miracles.'

My phone buzzed. It was my mother: *Just got your message.*

I'd texted her earlier about returning to London and said I was thinking seriously about dropping out of university.

You always finish things, she wrote.

Davika made a slurping sound so that her milkshake rattled a little.

I texted back: *I can't see any doctors in LA without insurance. Should I stay?*

A rush of wind knocked over a stack of styrofoam cups on the windowsill.

Davika waved her hand to say leave them.

My phone buzzed again: *Nathan. It's time.*

The room took on a grainy, dreamy aspect. My breathing grew sharp.

Davika guided me towards a chair and I sat down. She tried to distract me with a copy of *Vanity Fair*. I can't remember which actor was on the cover, maybe Angelina Jolie, but I stared at the image of her bare shoulders and thought they looked stuck on, like extra limbs that might have belonged to another actor, maybe Amy Adams. I sat there, lost in a Jolie/Adams mash-up, and said, 'Not right now,' and pushed the magazine away.

Her voice cracked with tenderness. 'I know you have to go.'

'What's wrong with me?'

'I wish I knew.' She smiled, sad and strained, and pulled me into her chest. 'I'll always be here.'

My mother: *I love you son.*

5

All is Strange to Me

It was early August and London was beautiful: sunbakers in parks, books in glass windows, baskets of fresh plums and beets at Borough Market, a crowd of punks eating ice cream outside the British Museum. At dusk, I picked leaves off the trees, then sorted them in my lap on the upper deck of buses. Green leaves, brown leaves, broken leaves. I wanted to carry pieces of the city around with me. The leaves were a reminder that nature was always present, even amid the sprawl and din.

I found a new flat and set about trying to study again. The drowning soldiers haunted me, but if I didn't manage to get back to my thesis, I was going to have to abandon it. Fees were mounting, debts growing larger by the day. My student loan was down to £33.10 – barely enough to scrape by for another couple of days. Resigned, I gritted my teeth and applied for another loan. Not long after, a fellow student connected me with a freelance job typing out complex equations for a postdoctoral researcher in the university's chemistry department. The pay was modest and the work monotonous, but it opened the door to similar opportunities, keeping me afloat for the time being.

My symptoms were often so painful that I slept all day, too exhausted to leave the house. Other days, when I was done with typing equations, I worked long hours on my thesis, hardly sleeping at all. Boom and bust.

The flat was chaos. Books piled up in rickety towers, many having fallen into heaps between clothes and boxes of vegetables and empty shopping bags. My living quarters looked like it had housed a drunken party, but, of course, there had been no party, only my inability to balance my illness with a clean room.

When I had the strength, I went for long walks, combing the clipped hedges of Kensington Gardens with my fingers, thinking about all the medical literature I'd read. I yearned to recover 'The Possibles' document. Surely the answer had been in there somewhere?

I told myself, *It's futile. No one has ever felt like this before.*

I couldn't have been more wrong. Throughout history, many people have suffered from depersonalisation. The first to write about it powerfully, and persuasively, was a nineteenth-century university professor from Geneva, Switzerland, Henri-Frédéric Amiel.

Although Amiel was a professor, he hated teaching, and was famous for giving the most boring lectures at the academy. He wrestled with why he was so bad at his job. Boring professors are commonplace, and they tend to write some variation on their thesis for their entire career. What held Amiel's fascination, and my own, was that he kept his own version of 'The Possibles' document. Overcome by depersonalisation, he took to the page to understand what ailed him, why he felt different from the people and the world around him. His private journal was published as *Journal Intime* after his death.

Over and over in its pages, Amiel returns to a feeling of unreality, detachment and terror. There was no escape for him. In its most infamous passage, he wrote a few lines that are now quoted by depersonalisation sufferers on internet forums and blogs: 'I find myself regarding existence as though from beyond the tomb, from another world. All is strange to me. I am, as it were, outside my own body and individuality; I am depersonalised, detached, cut adrift. Is this madness?' These lines were the first to name the illness, and to describe what it feels like in concise terms.

Like me, in pursuit of relief, Amiel went for long walks. Out in the fields, admiring the hawthorn and the roses, or sauntering up and down the Pont des Bergues under a moonlit sky, he would suddenly need a doctor. But even though he needed doctors often, they never seemed to help him. 'Why do doctors so often make mistakes?' he wrote. 'Because they are not sufficiently individual in their diagnoses or their treatment. They class a sick man under some given department, whereas every invalid is really a special case.' He thought that most doctors were close-minded and that they looked only for general patterns. 'Their methods of investigation are far too elementary.' Amiel imagined an ideal doctor who would have a profound knowledge of life and the soul, one who would be able to see intuitively what was causing the patient to suffer. Inevitably, he was let down – as many of us with mystery illnesses are – and became so frustrated by the incompetence of his doctors that he wondered if suicide might be a solution. It is a treatment after all, the final treatment. 'I have only wasted my time, my trouble, my money, and my hopes,' he wrote.

Because the illness remained a mystery to me, I shifted my hope of finding a diagnosis to longing, once again, for love. It was hard for me to give love, but I yearned to receive it in the belief it might alleviate the dark pain. A friend helped arrange several dates: breakfast with a curator who hated sugar, brunch with a marketing assistant who said her dream wedding would be in Somerset, a hole-in-the-wall taco place with an older woman who had two children and an ex-husband in jail for banking fraud.

The air was heavy. I had a secret: my illness.

One night, I went to a movie with an artist who painted abstract portraits and said things like, 'I hate technology,' and 'The best summers are in Provence.' It was late when we left the theatre. I was tired and silent. On a quiet street, she turned on me and said, 'There's something wrong with you,' which was very rude, but I couldn't disagree. I nodded my head and walked away.

My confidence was shattered.

Suddenly, every song on the radio was a lie.

I signed up to a popular dating site and filled out answers to questions about my hobbies and work history and desires. The process was endless. Boxes were ticked. With every new pop-up, it felt more invasive, and yet the site kept seducing me with the heads of women who swam across the screen like shiny fish. Were these names real? Marisa Boney, Natalie Hue, China Lott. Did someone called Sheila Manners really live on my street?

A cartoon smile appeared: *True Love Never Waits*.

There were four matches. Clicking on the profiles, I gasped – Maria's face was staring right at me. I did a double-take, then refreshed the page. What was she doing here? This was *my* site. I started writing her a private message but couldn't get my thoughts down on screen so I switched to writing in a notebook.

Maria,

My love for you means I can't stay silent. I am no good without you. Nothing in my life works without you. I believe deep down that you need me as much as I need you. I believe I can make you happy. I am willing to do the work and create a shared space for our love, a space of harmony and commitment. I believe this love will flourish and grow and become a life full of happiness. The past is behind us. We will be truly happy, like on that day when we stayed in bed for hours until the sun went down and you told me how much you loved to kiss me, how I felt like home. We can find that kiss again. We can find that lasting love. Do you believe we can? Are you willing to give it a chance? Not a minute passes without my being conscious of our love.

I typed this up and before pressing send, I added:

There is nobody else in the world. All the streets are empty. It's just you and me.

––––––

In his journal, Amiel is forever digressing. He describes landscapes and pieces of music, the light, the streets, the night, all of it rooted in philosophical questions about the nature of God, existence and the meaning of action. For all his musing on the divine, he always returns to his depersonalisation – the 'half-death' that had overtaken him.

His body feels inconsistent, vaporous, illusory. It has no gravity or solidity. He has no identity, no character, no individual nature. His self is lost. In one passage he writes that he doesn't recognise himself in the years gone by, that he is trapped in a cage without a self, perpetually turning around in search of it. In the end, he is nothing more than a reflection of two mirrors opposite one another.

What I find fascinating is that love was also a constant theme for Amiel. His desire for love became entangled with the mystery of his lost self. He thought love could make the self *visible* again and help him accept the passage of time. The love he needed was intense and powerful: 'I will have none of these passions of straw which dazzle, burn up, and wither ... I hope for the love which is great, pure and earnest, which lives and works in all the fibres.'

It was all or nothing. He wanted love at its highest point. This made for a life where he lurched wildly between highs and lows. He described himself as a shipwrecked sailor sinking beneath the waves. The water was always rising, the tides changing, the currents converging and rushing at his weak body, ready to pull him to the ocean floor and smother him in darkness. 'My soul is dying, my body is dying. In every direction the end is closing upon me.' The choice was profound: cling to life and swim, or give in to despair and drown.

For Amiel, true love was the link that could reunite the two parts of his self, the bridge to make him whole again. If he could grasp it, reality would no longer be in doubt, his vision clear, his fears forgotten, the knot of his struggles undone. Energy and concentration could return with the vigour of his youth, and he'd find the strength to embrace life again.

But such a need was not easily met. He was used to solitude and consumed by pain. When would this ideal love arrive? 'I am always waiting for the woman ... [who] shall be capable of taking entire possession of my soul, and of becoming my end and aim.'

From what I've learned, dating sites can also make you wait. They are a maze of buttons. You wait for your profile to upload, your photos to be approved. Choose your plan, enter your bank details, check your breathing, wait for the code in the confirmation email. Plug into the maze and steady your knees. If you wait, love is guaranteed. Every ten minutes a new couple falls in love.

The day after I messaged Maria, my phone rang from a blocked number. It was her, of course. I can't remember everything she said. She was so calm. I expected her to shout and tell me off, but she laid things out simply, 'I'm seeing other people now.'

Other people. As in, multiple? That floored me.

'You need to listen. This is the end.' She said this so quietly and firmly that her words seemed to stick to me. I knew she meant them.

No amount of trying to apologise or explain made any difference. Only one thing could have changed the course of things: if I was cured. Maybe then she would have agreed to meet again and discuss our fate. But my illness went unspoken, hovering between us on the line like a great black knot.

After she hung up, I felt impossible and gross, like trying to put dirty tissues back into the box. I thought of something she said to me when we first met, a quote from André Breton's novel *Nadja*: 'I will not go looking for keys.' She meant that when something was over, she wouldn't waste time thinking about it. She cut the cord for good. Whatever the reasons were, they no longer mattered. Her priority was the future – the next day, next season, next relationship.

I couldn't have been more different. For me, all the details were significant. I'd happily spend forever trying to piece them together and understand what happened.

Tell me why you didn't love me enough to nurture me in bad health, tell me why you never asked more questions instead of being angry with me because I didn't have the answers, tell me why you never believed I would get better, tell me why you left me behind on the steps to be alone with nothing but the unpaid gas bill.

Not only did I want to find the keys, but I needed Maria to place them in my hands and tell me exactly why my heart was so cold.

———

When we look at the history of depersonalisation, it becomes clear that doctors struggled with it long before Amiel began writing his journal. In the early nineteenth century, cases started piling up but no one knew what was happening. One Hungarian doctor was so frustrated by these strange new complaints that he called it The Baffling Thing. Patients all had comparable symptoms. In Stuttgart, Germany, a patient described having a complete lack of bodily sensations and believed he would be better off as a criminal – at least then he might experience a fear of death. Another, in Paris, said that an abyss lived between her body and the world; and another, at a French asylum, said she was neither dead or alive, but living in a continuous dreamworld of shadows and floating words.

One patient told his psychiatrist: 'Each of my senses, each

part of my proper self is as if it were separated from me and can no longer afford me any sensation. This impossibility seems to depend upon a void which I feel in the front of my head and to be due to a diminished sensibility over my whole body, for it seems to me that I never actually reach the objects that I touch. I no longer experience the internal feeling of the air when I breathe.'

These cases of The Baffling Thing prompted a search for what to call it. Doctors across Europe ruminated in journals and held conferences that erupted into heated debates. This debate continued for decades until, one morning in 1898, psychologist Ludovic Dugas discovered Amiel's journal and later published 'A Case of Depersonalisation', which formally introduced the term into the psychiatric literature.

The article focuses on a patient called M who has recently returned from a trip to Bath, in England. M begins to feel unwell. He encounters evening rain and wonders how the day preceding it was ever possible. He experiences midday as midnight and his memory disintegrates into fragments, detached from space and time: 'knowing neither when nor how his actions take place'. When M returns to France, the 'automatic acts' of his body take over his mind, causing him to feel a loss of self. Having read Amiel, Dugas immediately recognised M's experiences as symptoms of depersonalisation; it was a major breakthrough in the field of medicine.

Even though the illness baffled doctors more than a hundred years ago, it is a sad fact that when I returned to the clinic for help, no one could provide any answers. My blood was drawn. I did tests for liver and thyroid function. I had a chest x-ray and gave a stool sample to check my gut. When these came back normal, a doctor with a frog-like voice upped the dose of my existing medications: duloxetine, mirtazapine, olanzapine. She called it 'tweaking the cocktail', which made it sound like adding lime to a glass of gin, when it was actually a mind-altering surge of chemicals.

I distrusted the clinic, with its horrible track record for my case. Every new interaction seemed to make my illness worse and leave me more confused. Still, I took the pills and conjured enough energy to go for a run. Or so I thought. Halfway around the block, in new sneakers, the side effects hit, and I succumbed to waves of pain so great that before I could make it back inside, my bowel loosened and a blast of diarrhoea coursed down my legs.

In the toilet, I lay naked on the tiles and kept my body as straight as possible, which lessened the pain. Then I spent hours peeling the skin off grapes, filling bowl after bowl. Repeating the task was a welcome distraction. At the kitchen table, songs played in my mind. Old songs with strange melodies, songs of hope. I continued to believe that some doctor, somewhere, could put me on the right path. What other choice did I have but to keep returning to the clinic, asking questions, trying to articulate my trouble?

Amiel suffered in the same way. He felt humiliated by his doctors and was sceptical about everything they told him. He had two regular prescriptions, digitalis, now known as digoxin, taken orally or by injection for irregular heartbeat, and bromide, an anticonvulsant and sedative used to treat epilepsy. In his day, epilepsy was commonly thought to be caused by masturbation. In the eyes of the doctors, here was a lonely bachelor unable to stop soiling himself with pleasure. He was to be pitied, doped up with bromide, his sexual excitement reined in. But he was misdiagnosed, because we know from his journal that he wasn't interested in sex – he regarded it with disdain.

Although Amiel continued to take the drugs, they had no power over him, and he was left struggling: 'All possibilities are closed to me, one by one. It is difficult for the natural man to escape from a dumb rage against inevitable agony.' But he continued to try, knowing that 'in health there is liberty'.

If only he'd been able to get an appointment with Hyam Shorvon, a pioneering British psychiatrist who understood, as early as the 1940s, that depersonalised patients were not suffering from depression. Shorvon pioneered the treatment of trauma for soldiers after World War II. He used a method known as ether-induced abreaction, where through verbal suggestion, a patient has an unconscious reaction to a painful memory. The aim was to trigger a cathartic response.

In his paper 'A Depersonalisation Syndrome', Shorvon detailed his use of abreaction in treating patients with chronic depersonalisation. The results were convincing: many experienced a dramatic remission after just one session, while others showed varying levels of improvement. Based on this evidence, Shorvon concluded that depersonalisation was not a symptom, but an illness in its own right.

Although his approach never gained widespread adoption in mainstream psychiatry, Shorvon's work firmly established the illness in the medical literature. Indeed, he was the kind of doctor Amiel had dreamed of in his journal almost seventy years earlier.

Without adequate care of my own, chaos ensued when I could no longer contact Maria. As I walked to the dry cleaner, my mind dropped into its regular pattern of thinking about her, imagining what I would say, where the conversation would take place, under which sign, which lane, the time of day, what she'd be wearing, maybe the blue earrings.

But my mind corrected itself. I couldn't indulge this thinking any more. Her voice was strident: 'This is the end.' There was no ambiguity, no wiggle room.

Late at night, unable to sleep, I caught buses across the city and then waited in the rain for another one to take me back.

In those early hours, the wind was sour and biting. Something about being awake when most of the city was sleeping felt appropriate. It matched my dark emotions, living outside society, with no one to go home to and no one to love, swept along the streets of Vauxhall and Chigwell, Tooting and Wapping, Southwark and Aldgate, wondering what the next day would bring, how I'd go on.

One night I passed a billboard covered in giant numbers and got the idea to give out my phone number to strangers. I went to an all-night office-supply shop and made business cards. *Call me: 07947604211* They looked sharp – black and red. I handed them out to people, many of whom stared at me in disgust and dropped the card right in front of me. Some laughed in my face, while others kicked me in the shins and called me a 'fucking tourist'. The humiliation of the ritual became addictive. But sometimes people would take a card and thank me, saying it was a nice thing to do, to meet new people, especially in a city like London, which could be so lonely. I recognised in these faces something of my own pain, that they, too, were shouldering an invisible burden and needed the company of others.

The problem was no one ever called me. Despite giving out hundreds of cards – nothing. I started lurking in the streets around Kingsway and saw walls of tart cards inside the phone boxes. The nudes dared me to call ('English Lass Wants To

Bang', 'Romp All Night With Trans Swede Lucy', 'Busty Scot Wants Your Sauce'). Instead, I took them down and put my own cards up. In contrast to the glossy images, mine was mysterious, floating above the phone like a secret prize.

Most of the people who called wanted to talk dirty, but one sex worker, who went by Brenda Lee, yelled at me for taking down her card and said I owed her £10,000 for a week in lost earnings.

Did she really make that much? 'Sod off.'

One guy called to tell me he was homeless, another said he'd lost his job, and a banker in town from America wanted me to come to his suite and talk about 'liquid assets'. The end of my experiment came when I heard non-stop sobbing. This call was different. Somebody was in real distress. He didn't want to give his name but said he'd called my number because he'd tried the Suicide Helpline and couldn't get through. He was alone. His room was bitterly cold. He couldn't get warm. No amount of extra clothing or blankets was of any help. For weeks he'd been unable to sleep and was growing desperate. His family were useless. Life wasn't what he wanted it to be. Turning forty was horrible. There was one good summer when he was young but the rest were a blur of bad relationships and signing on for benefits. The high street used to be booming but now all the shops were boarded up. Everyone had moved away.

Each time I tried to reassure the man, he thought I was trying to get off the call and would beg me to stay with him. 'I need you,' he said. 'I can't do this without you.' We talked for hours, two lost souls, awake in the dark, and before the man hung up, he said, 'I want to live. I want to see the sun.' He promised to call again, but days later I changed my number. It was all too much.

———

With my longing to recover 'The Possibles' document, what I didn't know was that there was a book that could have helped me: *The Diagnostic and Statistical Manual of Mental Disorders* (the *DSM*). Known as the bible of psychiatrists, it is a controversial guide intended to support mental health diagnoses. In the first edition, published in 1952, depersonalisation was only a symptom within the broader category of disassociation. It was later upgraded to a disorder in its own right, but with a caveat that some doctors questioned its inclusion. When the latest edition (*DSM-5*) came out in 2013, even the then director of the National Institute of Mental Health in the US, Thomas Insel, said the book was 'no longer sufficient for researchers'.

People with depersonalisation often complain about the *DSM* because of its vague and watered-down criteria for the illness. For such a doorstopper, at close to 1000 pages, the book is hardly a manual for depersonalisation. Only a few pages are dedicated to the illness, which read like a compromise between warring factions. But for all the *DSM*'s flaws, it does offer a basic description of the symptoms that those suffering from depersonalisation can recognise:

— The individual may feel detached from his or her entire being (e.g. 'I am no one,' 'I have no self')
— There may also be a diminished sense of agency
(e.g. feeling robotic, like an automaton; lacking control of one's speech or movements) ... one of a split self, with one part observing and one participating
— Individuals may suffer extreme rumination or obsessional preoccupation (e.g. constantly obsessing about whether they really exist, or checking their perceptions to determine whether they appear real)
— Individuals with depersonalisation ... may have difficulty describing their symptoms and may think they are 'crazy' or 'going crazy'.

What I find difficult to square is that doctors themselves are largely ignorant, or at odds with, the *DSM*'s criteria. Although the book is dense with technical information and contains hundreds of specific diagnoses, it's shocking that depersonalisation remains widely misdiagnosed when an accurate explanation is readily available. Remarkably, the basic description of symptoms is consistent with Amiel's account of his illness. The professor could never have imagined that his private journal, unpublished at the time of his death, would go on to become a crucial text in the history of mental health.

But even though Amiel wrote about his illness, it didn't help him receive an accurate diagnosis or treatment. The words were on the page, yet he remained sick. This is also true of the *DSM*. Despite the inclusion of depersonalisation, because of the book's controversial status, it is often left to gather dust, leaving patients misdiagnosed. In my view, we need to fundamentally rethink the *DSM* and combine symptom-based categories with behavioural and neuroscientific evidence. Doing so will allow clinicians to see the different studies associated with the illness and make an assessment based on accurate and up-to-date findings. Any print version of the *DSM* becomes outdated almost immediately. To address this and make the manual more dynamic, it should be available online. This would allow medical professionals to add new, critical information following a peer-review process.

———

From across the classroom, it was as if a force flowed between us, a strange magnetism. We noticed each other right away. I saw on her face, and in the hunch of her shoulders, that she knew great sadness – she saw it in me too. The lecturer was talking about Rodin's sculptures, or maybe Paul Klee. Autumn sun poured through the windows. She was in her early sixties and wore a necklace of colourful stones. The Friday-afternoon lectures were open to the public, but until now I'd only ever seen students. Although there was a notebook in her lap, the woman didn't seem to be listening, and every minute or so she pulled out a tissue and toyed with it in her hands. When we caught one another's eye, she turned away and waited, before locking eyes with me again.

My heart began to beat. Had we met before? Who was she?

After the lecture, I retreated to the student bar, where she approached me and ordered a round of sandwiches and pilsners. It was as if we'd arranged to meet – old friends. But she was a stranger. Her name was Angela Bass. She had penetrating blue eyes. At first I couldn't pick the accent, but soon learned she was from the Canadian prairies in Alberta.

'Cowboy country,' she said. 'Tough place.'

Our connection was instant. I didn't want her to stop talking. Each snapshot of her life drew me further in. Western Canada could be violent, she said, especially for women who grew up in small towns with fathers too fond of the bottle.

London was better, a gateway to the world. She loved art and art history, especially the Austrian Expressionist painter Egon Schiele, and thought my PhD thesis sounded better than the lecture we'd endured. When last drinks was called, she fingered her necklace and said she lived nearby in Bedford Square.

Her house was a large terrace full of plants and heavy carpet. Paintings hung salon-style. She gave me a tour. On the staircase, we stopped in front of a small landscape by the Impressionist Alfred Sisley. The way she lingered over it, leaning into its frame, pointing at the little stone bridge, showed me how much it meant to her.

'I bought it after my husband died, when I first got to London.'

We sat in a room full of exquisite furniture and rich wallpaper. In the middle of her coffee table was an old anthology: *The Big Book of Family Poetry*. She took off her jumper and made a show of pouring scotch into heavy glasses. We drank a few. She put on a record, but it was a terrible old classical recording with too many violins and we ended up laughing and changing the record to one with a woman's voice from the 1950s who sang about going to heaven. What a mystery: to sit in the dark with a charming companion.

'What did you do before you retired?'

'I helped my husband with the oil business,' she said, tugging at a strand of her brittle hair. 'He never meant to beat me. Or maybe he did. I hated him for many years, but somehow I was still devastated when he died. It doesn't really make sense.'

'Maybe it doesn't have to.'

She sank back into the lounge. 'What's your greatest fear?'

We were in such a flow I didn't hesitate. 'Having a bath.'

She never asked why, and I didn't have to explain. The reason didn't matter. Somehow, she understood. I was so comfortable in her presence that it was like meeting a long-lost relative. Our blood felt the same.

'Okay,' she said, and after finishing her glass, took me gently by the hand, like a mother does to a child, and walked me down the hall into her bathroom. She ran a bath, and when it was high and full of soapy water, she sat in a chair. I took off my clothes and lowered myself in. My body – the animal. She looked on in silence. I sniffed the soap and felt a great pressure at the back of my head.

The low light closed in around me.

I howled, a cry of pain that erupted into a throttle.

She leaned over and said quietly, 'There's no use in any of that,' before patting me on the head, over and over, until I was calm. She then lifted my feet out and buried her face in them, massaging her wrinkled cheeks against my toes. The bones of my feet met the bones of her face. She sobbed wet, heavy tears, her breath warm on my skin. Her mascara smudged, trickling into the sides of her mouth.

'My dear boy,' she kept saying. 'My dear, dear boy ...'

I got dressed and we lay holding each other on the lounge. She gripped me so tightly I thought I'd never get to sleep, but with all my crying I was exhausted, and passed out to the *tick-tick* of the record player.

In the morning I woke and felt, like Amiel, that the day had 'something of the night' clinging to it. Heading home on the bus, with the city coming alive around me, I was overcome by the feeling of being violently understood by another person, a chance meeting of intense belonging – the kind of connection I'd hoped for when handing out my number to strangers.

I thought of the bridge in her painting, how it floated above the stairs and how she pointed to it, and said, 'What a beautiful place to cross over.'

6

The Burning Question

February is the most depressing month in London. Christmas decorations have finally come down, the bank balance is in the red, and the weather is bleak enough to be the envy of goths around the world. The fog gets into your pores. On the train, in the off-licence, or at the post office, people shake out umbrellas and tell stories about food banks and rising crime.

In the corner of the pharmacy, you hear complaints about the price of medication and how the city is full of empty houses while so many Londoners sleep rough. The problem is globalism, or something about taxes and pain. If it's an especially rough day, you might even hear a student quote Philip Larkin: *Among the rain and stone places / I find only an ancient sadness falling / Only hurrying and troubled faces.*

Amid this atmosphere, I longed to be back with Angela in Bedford Square. We'd become fast friends after our first night together, seeing plays, movies and a memorably grand performance of Wagner's *Das Rheingold* at the Royal Opera House. We drank so much lapsang tea that she joked we might go up in smoke. But she travelled a lot and was now at her house in Spain, as she was every winter. She sent me photos of her reading by the pool. We tried talking on the phone but I knew she hated her 'stupid little device'. After the intimacy of being in person, it just wasn't the same.

Before she left London, I told her in detail about my illness and the search for a cure. She offered money, whatever she could do. I said I'd done everything. Money wouldn't help, not at this stage.

'You think of this thing you have as forever,' she said. 'But I've lived long enough to know that there are just these bad seasons in life. Sometimes these seasons go on for years, decades even. And then one day, maybe when you're out getting groceries, you get a call to say your husband is dead and it's over. The world is new again.'

With Angela gone, the winter hit hard, and I struggled to find new ways to cope. She sent me a leather-bound notebook with a sturdy spine and I wrote 'Possible Joys' on the cover. It wasn't a question of finding my true illness, not any more. Now, with no new leads, I put my search aside. Just as I had done with 'The Possibles' document, I began organising lists of activities into four columns.

1/ Games 2/ Music 3/ Movies 4/ Beyond.

I furiously added items as if preparing for the apocalypse. When I tried something that wasn't joyful, I crossed it off:

Meg Ryan

~~Tetris~~

Fellini

Burial's *Untrue*

~~watercolours~~

Liz Phair

~~Solitaire~~

~~Beethoven~~

~~Requiem for a Dream~~

Basquiat

I tried doing second-hand jigsaws of grand country houses but could never finish them. There were always a few pieces missing. One morning I found an old DVD copy of the Woodstock documentary lying next to some bins on the street. I watched it on repeat, getting lost in the crowds and grimy riffs. In one of the notorious hippie scenes, couples swim naked in the midday sun, paddling and laughing. Others run in from the bank to join them, humming and singing, circling one another. The grainy footage was Eden. Forget Vietnam and the assassinations, forget the Manson murders. Swim out to us – this afternoon will go on forever.

The water was a space of sheer joy. I watched the swimmers again and again, reliving their smiles. Would I ever be so happy in the water? Was it possible to be so free?

This reverie was a distraction from the burning question: What caused me to become so sick? The visceral night of my onset was clear, but what was the cause? One of the many harrowing things about depersonalisation is that it's difficult to pin down exactly what brings it about.

My assumption was that the acute stress of my graduate study, insecure work, intense relationship with Maria, and the night swimming incident – as the catalyst – all had something to do with it. Still, it was hard to believe these circumstances, however challenging, were sufficient to explain my dark pain and loss of self. But science suggests that in many patients it is precisely these sustained, lower-level experiences – what psychologists colloquially call little-'t' traumas – that can trigger an onset.

What I find incredible is that the very notion of little-'t' traumas redefines how we think of trauma. In her book *Trauma and Recovery*, psychiatrist Judith Herman challenges the view that trauma is limited to single, catastrophic events – earthquakes, car accidents, combat, terrorist attacks or witnessing the murder of a loved one. Instead, sustained stresses can amount to chronic trauma, much like how for soccer players, years of heading the ball, rather than one severe concussion, can result in the brain disorder CTE. Unlike stress, trauma lingers. The dark pain doesn't pass, it burrows deep, settling within.

Dr Emma Černis, a clinical psychologist at the University of Birmingham, says the mind's repeated use of dissociation as a protective mechanism can lead to it becoming a default escape. The body moves beyond the initial fight-or-flight response that we commonly associate with anxiety, and into a dissociative state. For those of us with depersonalisation, when the brain realises it's trapped, a switch is flipped. The build-up of small-scale triggers and rising anxiety then becomes a learned, over-rehearsed response – a fixed state of unreality.

While the notion of sustained, minor traumas makes sense in my case, dramatic events like physical abuse in childhood – big-'T' trauma – also make a person predisposed to depersonalisation, whose onset may occur years after the abuse took place. At this point, often during adolescence or early adulthood, psychological defences are severely impaired. It's not difficult to imagine how the experience of such abuse might make someone feel as if the world is unreal, or fixate on birth and mourn their lost self.

One patient, a woman living in Bucharest, Romania, was violently beaten by her stepfather during childhood. She reached out to her mother but was told: 'You must respect your stepfather.' Many years later, at age twenty, the woman developed chronic depersonalisation, floating outside her apartment to escape reality. She also spoke in a baby-like voice, desperately wanting to go back to a time before the trauma took hold, before her sense of self was lost.

For depersonalised patients who have been violently raped, many describe how during the assault they managed to 'escape' their bodies by floating above the scene and observing from a distance. This transient experience of depersonalisation then becomes chronic when they cannot resume normal life and remain trapped outside their body.

A 25-year-old American woman raped by three strangers one Thanksgiving was struck down by depersonalisation afterwards: 'The wasteland limbo in which I currently reside is a world between worlds, where I wait to be born.' Her life became emotionally disconnected, unreal and impermanent. At the time of her assault, the patient was very close to finishing her PhD. But when she became depersonalised, it ended her study for good.

———

Going back to my Possible Joys notebook, I decided on something from the Beyond column, which was a menagerie of ambitious or hare-brained ideas. I was fascinated by a Rubens painting, *The Elevation of the Cross*, and thought of reconstructing it in tiny pieces of coloured paper. The painting has dramatic contrasts of dark and light, an abundance of clean skin, and a sheep dog who's drunk on the action. Christ's loincloth, too, seems to be falling off. It's intricate, provocative, kitsch, sexy, and a celebration of the physical body. Most importantly, it was complicated enough to be a real challenge to complete.

I bought a trolley full of coloured paper, traced the outline of the painting onto a giant piece of cardboard, and, laying it out on the floor, began gluing down tiny pieces.

Before long, I was immersed, and this Possible Joy was on its way to becoming an Actual Joy. But I fell into a trap when I began to contemplate the original painting. Here was a dying man, his soul squinting, his mind in dark corners, everything in the world against him, his security, his comfort, his calling. He was being raised up only to die. Something about the mystery of the painting made me think I would never know the cause of my illness, never answer the question about my lost sense of self. And this terrified me. I couldn't accept not knowing. There must be an answer, something still hidden from me.

In the week leading up to Easter, I spent time in the quiet confines of the Brompton Oratory. The church smelt of incense and wood polish. Statues were covered in purple fabric for Lent. I wanted to uncover them, tracing their folds with my eyes. The way the veils bunched up reminded me of all the robes in the painting, and I marvelled at how Rubens was able to capture the crucifixion in such vivid detail.

I got talking to a priest about John Henry Newman, the English theologian who helped found the church. He recommended Newman's book *Apologia Pro Vita Sua* – which translates as *A Defence of One's Own Life* – and said the novelist Muriel Spark converted to Catholicism after reading it. I found an old paperback copy on Charing Cross Road and read long into the night. My experience of its pages was an extension of the Oratory itself: rich, baroque and mysterious. Newman quoted himself constantly, sifting through old sermons, thoughts and memories.

One morning, in 1833, he was struck down by typhoid fever, certain he would die: 'I sat down on my bed, and began to sob violently.' His servant Gennaro asked for any final words, at which point Newman became determined to live: 'I shall not die, for I have not sinned against light.' He struggled with how to become whole again, to regain his sense of self: 'I wish to be known as a living man, and not as a scarecrow which is dressed up in my clothes.'

Newman helped make sense of why I was drawn to the Rubens painting – to focus on Christ's suffering, not my own. Piecing the mosaic together, in my amateurish way, was a means of surrendering my pain to a narrative, an ancient story of faith and human struggle. One I knew well. My mosaic was huge. Maybe 10,000 pieces of paper. The result, however, wasn't fit to be seen. Christ looked stilted, kid-like, abstract. But I liked that it was so bad. The simplicity humbled the grandeur of the painting and made Christ's suffering more accessible to me.

———

The fact that there is a direct link between marijuana and depersonalisation is not widely known. In recent years, as the drug has become legal in states across the US – and Canada – there have been many positive benefits, including reducing the decades of disproportionate harm suffered by communities of colour, who were unfairly targeted under previous drug laws. Many people were given harsher sentences and were more likely to be incarcerated than their white counterparts. Legalisation has not only begun to rectify this injustice but also provided opportunities for these communities to participate in the legal cannabis industry. But increased access has a serious downside. Teenagers are most at risk because the distribution of cannabinoid receptors (CB1) in the adolescent brain is not always the same as in the adult brain; the tracts of white matter containing CB1 are still developing. This means that intoxication for young people is typically stronger and, for many, prolonged.

Kari Franson, a professor of clinical pharmacy at the University of Southern California, says marijuana use can lead to abnormal circuitry in the brain. Whether the drug is smoked or consumed in edibles, marijuana triggers depersonalisation, sending many teenagers to the emergency room, where their stomachs are pumped to reduce toxicity. At this stage it can be too late. In one study at Mount Sinai Hospital in New York, fifteen out of 117 patients (13 per cent) reported a clear and immediate onset of depersonalisation after smoking marijuana, from which they never returned to their normal state.

One eighteen-year-old girl said that after getting sober she was in class at high school and felt invisible, like a fictional character. She was plagued by alternative-reality thoughts and saw herself as a large bird. One seventeen-year-old boy presented to the emergency department a week after smoking a bong saying that he was living outside his body. After no organic etiology was identified, he was sent home. His grades suffered dramatically, and although he appeared normal to others, he remained depersonalised for months.

For this book, I've spoken to many teenagers who describe themselves as ghosts, one of whom compared his illness to the movie adaptation of Charles Dickens' *A Christmas Carol*. After smoking marijuana, he felt like a ghost lost in time, drifting between the past, present and future. But unlike the movie, his altered state never ended. Another boy identified with Lydia Deetz, the character played by Winona Ryder in *Beetlejuice*, when she talks about living in a dark room.

When I was speaking on the phone to a girl named Prue Welch, who fell ill with depersonalisation after smoking marijuana in the mountains of Utah, she gave me this warning: 'Never watch that movie *Mother!* with Jennifer Lawrence, the one where she sees a heart living in the walls. It made my symptoms so much worse. I already feel like my life is a movie, and watching *Mother!* put me in so much more hell. I feel like people with depersonalisation should be very careful about what we look at. And that movie – holy shit! It was all nightmares.'

Drugs like ecstasy, LSD and ketamine are also known to provoke an onset of depersonalisation. Although many people use these substances without it resulting in illness, research suggests that some patients are more biologically vulnerable due to factors such as genetic predisposition, pre-existing mental health conditions or underlying neurological differences. In these cases, the drugs initiate a potent chemical trigger that distorts – and then disrupts – key pathways in the brain, potentially leading to long-term changes in functioning. One study found that seven out of forty patients (17.5 per cent) who used these drugs developed chronic depersonalisation. Another found that 97 out of 608 patients (16 per cent) had an onset of the illness. Both studies highlight that a significant minority of users, particularly those with pre-existing vulner-abilities, are affected.

Researchers use the concept of a tipping point to explain such cases. Imagine the brain as a river with many currents. For a boat to sail smoothly, these currents must remain balanced. However, in those who are biologically predisposed, the drugs disrupt this balance, causing the currents to collapse and the boat to crash onto the rocks.

'I felt like the person I was before had been entirely wiped from all sense memory,' said one patient a month after using LSD, 'and I felt completely dissociated from the body I was inhabiting. I essentially felt like I was completely disintegrating. My life has and never will be the same.'

———

After my Rubens mosaic and reading John Henry Newman, I was flush with religious feeling. Lying in bed, I thought about paradise – the word. The first half, *para*, was so singular, full of direction, while *dise* expanded outwards, a tumbling throw of the dice. Paradise comes from the Greek *paradeisos*, meaning an idyllic place, often associated with a heavenly garden. Paradise is the opposite of hell, a place of light. I wanted that, *needed* it. Lift me into the light away from my illness.

Is that choral music?

The appeal of paradise is that it comes after suffering. We don't begin life in the garden. We have to experience the pain of life in order to reach paradise. It's the other side of illness, a place with no need for doctors or clinics. No need for medicine. When Rubens painted Christ on the cross, he asked us to imagine paradise outside the borders of the painting. He showed us that mortal pain is the only way into the garden.

I thought of the full-bodied person I once was and tried to recall some Actual Joys, glimpses of paradise on earth:

— The feel of driving an old Toyota across a muddy field days after I first got my licence.

— The taste of water that came out of the garden hose near the strawberry patch on my grandmother's farm.

— The first pages of Thomas Hardy's *Tess of the d'Urbervilles*.

— The way starlings fly in formation.

— The sight of a newborn calf in the dusk.

— The sound of Jeff Buckley on the car radio in 1997.

— The moment at sunset after I climbed a hill in
Switzerland as a fresh-faced backpacker and looked back
at the city of Bern, thinking no, there could be no more
sublime a sight, only to hear the church bells come on,
one by one.

My room was small, my sheets crumpled. I was meant to be
reading for my PhD but ended up reading something different: a biography of the German poet Heinrich Heine. A friend
pushed it on me, saying Heine suffered from a mysterious
illness. On a midday hike, the poet was struck down, never
able to walk again. Half-blind, he was confined to his house in
agony. Morphine was no help. His room was filled with piles
of mattresses, allowing him to stretch and wriggle around.

He wrote to his brother Maximilian, a doctor, and said
he was now confined to a mattress grave: 'This living death,
this half-life, is unbearable, especially with so much pain.' In
this life-and-death struggle, Heine looked God in the eye and
knew there was only one thing to do – keep working. Between
bouts of hallucination and vomiting, Heine produced the
most searing and intimate poetry of his life.

What a strange experience to read about this sick poet
while I was also confined to bed. The page in front of me
was only half in focus and the author was describing Heine's

extraordinary strength in being able to write his poems while rolling and coughing in his mattress grave: 'I have a double, another poor wretch that is coupled to me. He looks so sick and wretched, so pale and emaciated. He looks at me with painful scorn and thereby strangely unnerves me. The fellow maintains he is I myself, that the two of us are only one person, that we are one single wretched man now suffering ... my damned second self.'

I was half absorbing the words on the page but also drifting off to worry about my own mysterious illness, and how I really didn't want to go blind or be stuck in a mattress grave, when I read that Heine also thought about paradise. For him, it was a landscape of palm trees and ocean scent. All he wanted was relief from his body's despair, to be at the end of his illness, cured of pain: 'I must leave all that made the world so precious.'

When you are stuck in bed reading about paradise there is a natural urge to put the book down and type the word into a search engine. You might find a hotel with the name, or a clothing brand, maybe a pop song. The online dictionary will tell you that paradise is 'heaven, the final abode of the righteous'. There are also images, lots of them, and you don't have to scroll too far to find the most common paradise on the internet: porn. So many porn stars have the name Paradise that it's difficult to tell them apart. *Click here.* Wild paradise, orgy in paradise, blondes in paradise, beards in paradise – acres of digital flesh.

One cause of depersonalisation that has become increasingly prevalent is porn addiction, especially among teenagers. Watching hours of Sasha Paradise, Ken Paradise, Christine Paradise, or any other porn star performing hardcore sex acts, can severely disrupt healthy psychological development. Pleasure is more easily absorbed when it's exaggerated, and the brain becomes conditioned to seek the intense dopamine rush that porn offers. Over time, teenagers begin to prioritise this rush over real-life interaction, leading to an onset of depersonalisation. While this may be transient at first, it becomes chronic when the significance of the physical body diminishes.

It is a paradox. Although the individual must engage the physical body to immerse themselves in the screen, depersonalisation sets in when the body becomes merely a tool – an automaton – serving the screen's demands rather than its own needs. The cliché is: With enough rope, a man will hang himself. Here, with a pornography addiction, the body gradually fades away, becoming complicit in its own erasure.

One patient, a 21-year-old with a serious porn addiction, described himself as a zombie: 'I've battled depersonalisation so bad it's not even funny. I've been to the lowest I've ever been. I've lived an existence that has been pure hell on earth ...

Real-life girls don't interest me at all.' The only way back to reality was a complete detox from the screen, in which he told himself: 'Don't touch your dick unless you're pissing or washing it. No questions, just don't.'

During the COVID-19 pandemic, there was an exponential rise in cases of digital depersonalisation, which psychologists described as being 'Zoomed out'. As early as March 2020, worldwide internet use increased by nearly 70 per cent, and Zoom usage increased by a factor of ten. Whether it was for school, work, doctor appointments, ballet recitals, birthdays or funerals, everyone was on Zoom. The gallery view, where bodies appear like baseball cards on a single screen, overwhelms our central vision, which is crucial for maintaining focus. This makes it difficult to meaningfully process any one person. Digital bodies, in this view, are always incomplete, often blurry, and subject to frequent disruptions.

A student who missed the freedom and authenticity of being taught in person developed symptoms while in lockdown: 'I feel like a strange copy of me is participating in a Zoom class, while another me is watching this from the side. It's like in a dream. As if I need to wake up to get myself back.'

Zoom is not the only piece of software that puts people at risk of depersonalisation. The rapid growth of virtual reality (VR) has also led to an uptick in cases. VR headsets, like Apple's Vision Pro and Google's Daydream View, immerse users in an unreal world. Much of digital culture relies on masks: avatars, emojis and filtered selfies. But these headsets are *literal* masks that plug into an alternative reality.

Take, for example, the popular video game *Skyrim*. In a dark, embattled landscape, you carry a sword, wear armour and battle dragons while running through dungeons. Your task is to defeat the World-Eater. While on your quest, feel free to forget your car payments, student debt, overdue rent and the stomach ache you have from eating too much dark chocolate. While a game like this might, at first, seem too fantastical or silly to compete with the real world, a recent study conducted by the Department of Psychiatry at the University of Bonn in Germany found that otherwise healthy participants developed transient depersonalisation symptoms after playing *Skyrim* for short periods with a VR headset. The game's *unreality* was so powerful it left participants uncertain about their body and environment.

As this technology grows and becomes even more immersive, researchers like Frederick Aardema, who directs a mental health laboratory at the University of Montreal, Canada, are sounding the alarm, pointing to evidence that even a single VR session can lead to symptoms. 'The feeling of immersion, whether physical or psychological in nature, allows the user to either feel or believe that he or she has left the real world,' Aardema explains. This disconnection can fundamentally alter our sense of self, blurring the line between the simulated and the real to an extent that the brain struggles to reconcile.

Spending hours using VR without interruption can significantly increase the risk of depersonalisation. To mitigate this harm, it's important to limit VR exposure time and take regular breaks to recalibrate the senses. This is especially critical for young people, whose developing brains are more vulnerable to the disorienting effects of prolonged engagement. However, the responsibility does not rest with users alone. The tech industry must take an active role in safeguarding the risk of depersonalisation, and mental health more broadly, by designing systems with built-in time limits, periodic reminders to pause, and tools to help users reconnect with their physical surroundings. Without these measures, we risk allowing VR's transformative potential to overshadow its psychological consequences. Rather than viewing VR as mere entertainment, we should treat it as a tool with profound effects on perception, much like a powerful drug that requires careful regulation.

Current consensus among behavioural scientists indicates that by 2030 we will spend more time in simulated digital environments than in the physical world. With this profound shift in our way of life, depersonalisation cases are expected to increase dramatically.

———

Angela sent me a text to meet her at the Whitechapel Gallery. She was back from Spain. After building my stamina for several weeks with short walks, I felt ready for my first night out in months. The exhibition was full of framed pieces of fabric, and small sculptures made of LEGO and balsa wood. Over a glass of wine, Angela said she had a gift for me: an old book about Goya. I fingered its spine and marvelled at its end-papers. She kissed me on the cheek, and said, 'Only for you.'

Out on the pavement, as she was telling me about the dusty antique shop where she bought the book in Cordoba, there was a massive bang across the street.

Two bodies, flying through the air. A man and a woman.

The jeep was bent against a barrier, its bonnet crumpled in. Windows shattered. Headlights smashed. For a split second: silence.

I started to run, glass crunching under my shoes. People began pointing and waving their hands and one woman holding a baby screamed at the sight of the crash and the raw terror in her voice brought people out of shops and cafes to cover their mouths in horror. Many of us in the crowd were running together, converging on the bodies, yelling at pedestrians to get back.

'Someone call an ambulance.'

'They're not moving.'

'His head is bleeding.'

'Lift his arm over.'

'What can we do? Look at them.'

'He's only a boy.'

'I think they're a couple.'

'Take off your shirt. Try wrapping it around.'

'Cover the —'

'Get out of the way.'

'Don't try and lift her. We have to wait.'

'There's nothing you can do.'

A plume of black smoke shot out of the jeep.

'No, it was two cars.'

'They were racing.'

'But I saw —'

'The jeep lost control.'

'Try the number again. We have to get through.'

'Christ, was he —'

'Jane. Cover your eyes. Don't look at her. Come over here. *Don't look at her, I said.*'

'She can't see.'

'That's all I know.'

'Don't say that. If you're not here to help —'

'Turn him over.'

'We have to wait for the ambulance.'

'Fuck.'

'They can't get through.'

'It's a crime scene.'

'We don't have a choice.'

A small white dog leapt out of a woman's handbag and ran up and down the pavement, jumping over the bodies while the woman ran after it shouting, 'Samson! Samson, don't do that!'

The dog stopped barking and licked the hand of the man on the ground.

The man wasn't moving.

Police and ambulance drove up on the pavement as frenzied hands waved them down and others grew scared they might be run over and criss-crossed the street to shelter and look on. Sirens pierced the air as medics surrounded the bodies.

'We need a spinal collar, and bring the monitor.'

'Count to three. Ready? One, two …'

'When I say GO.'

'It's not working.'

'She can't talk, her skull's cracked. You can see the veins there.'

'What's her name?'

'Focus on me. We're here to help.'

'The scene isn't secure.'

'Our Father. Who art in heaven.'

'We're right here, love.'

Rain started falling over the street.

Captain, there are no more boats.

'Pass me the bandage.'

'We're running out of time.'

'He's not responding. There's no response.'

You heard the order. Abandon ship. We need to swim.

But the Germans —

Honking, rumbling, screeching.

'Excuse me, sir. My name is Constable Hargreave. Did you see the accident?'

Angela came to stand with me in the rain. We held each other and cried as they loaded the bodies then sped away to the hospital. There was a bare feeling in the atmosphere and the few birds above, which had been playful, made no sound. Leaves fell through the air.

On the way home we sat next to each other in a near-empty train carriage and listened to music, one earbud each. David Bowie's voice pressed into my brain. I kept replaying the sight of the bodies and thought how easily it could have been me lying on the pavement. The jeep came so close, maybe ten metres away. Seeing a man of my age on the ground like that brought back the days I'd spent on the balcony, wanting to jump. This is what it would have looked like, I thought. Limbs buckled, broken, elbows torn, a gash in the neck, blood leaking into the gutters.

The man's body was my body. The man's face was my face.

The medic was talking about me when he said, 'There's no response.'

The next morning, still reeling from what I'd seen, my symptoms were unbearable. I sat cross-legged on the kitchen floor, cursing my second self, cursing the doctors and the medical establishment. This was never going to end. What was I to do but shuffle along to yet another doctor and specialist and tired nurse? What was I to do but continue down the same brick path to the next clinic, the next referral? My nightmares are full of your high-back chairs and tweed jackets – You could have helped me – What did you expect of me, to crawl into the clinic dripping in blood and shit? What could I have possibly done differently with my little speech and mortal hands? Where were the friendly doctors I'd heard so much about in newspaper columns? Where were the specialists who stayed longer after hours neglecting their own families to read newly published studies ready to give the gift of knowledge to their profession and save that one extra life, that one extra human head at the dinner table who could eat their fucking beans and ice cream with hope in their heart and knowledge that the day's new dawn would be brighter on the flowers? Was it too abstract for you? Was it too crude, too weird? What was happening? All I gave you in my hope and my language – I fought for you people to understand me, every day I fought with everything I had to stay off the high balcony on my tiptoes looking down at the great asphalt. I fought with every breath I had, sucking everything I could out of the air in my horrid little lounge room, gasping again and again at the knowledge that eluded me – Don't you fucking read? It was there on the shelf. All you needed to do was reach for the book and turn to the contents page. I know, I know. It's a labyrinth. Stop blathering for one goddamn minute about *mental health* and start listening to what I am actually saying. All I needed was a few extra minutes of your time – But no – Never enough time, always the next patient, next in line, not enough government money, still more work to be done, more research needed, more meetings, more consultants, so many benefits and answers but not here in this clinic, with its smell of bad deli meat and antiseptic, not for me sitting for another hour closer to the end of the night – I grabbed at the air, hopeless, not going on, and yet going on, but where were you?

My phone pinged with a message.

Ever since my symptoms began, my mother, who lived in Sydney, had occasionally tried to help in the search for a diagnosis by sending links to local doctors. Often these were accompanied by a plea for me to get on a plane to Australia. Most of the doctors looked wholesome, with neat collars and high necklines – straight from central casting. Nothing to suggest they would be any better than doctors in the UK.

But something about the doctor's face in this new message spoke to me. The intense way he looked down the camera gave me a sense he might be different. His details were impressive: thirty years working with patients as a clinical psychologist, publishing studies and advising government bodies. I was intrigued, but experience taught me to be sceptical.

Another ping. My mother had made me an eCard. There was a whale and a Bible quote, from Jonah: 'The waters closed in over me to take my life; the deep surrounded me; weeds were wrapped around my head. I called out to the Lord, out of my distress, and he answered me.'

7

Two Lights

The garage was small. I couldn't believe it had ever fit a Mitsubishi Sigma. At the edge of a window with poor trims, a warm breeze sliced in. Boxes of toys and garden supplies propped up a bicycle with flat tyres. The tag on a crumpled nylon bag said 'Two Man Tent'. Stacks of old magazines sat on top of tote bags with holes in the corners, while failed scholarship applications peered ominously from a filing cabinet.

In London, I had no money, no job, no strength to study, few friends and very little hope I'd ever get better. I didn't know how to go on and felt I had little choice but to live with my mother, at least for the time being. The garage was built for a car to come and go, to be free on the roads. But it was now a place I came to be still and try to recover.

After a long and sleepless flight from Heathrow to Sydney, the taxi ride deep into the suburbs was the slowest ride of my life. The wide lawns and the windows of TV light appeared to be laughing at me, low and dark.

I was trying to assemble a foldout bed. Suitcases were strewn across the garage floor, clothes spilling out. My mother appeared at the door in her blue cardigan, squinting at me as she ate salted cashews, one by one, from a plastic container. 'You might be able to finally get better here,' she said. 'You never know. This could be it.'

'I'll try and get some sleep. That's all that matters right now.'

'It's not that bad in here.' She glanced quickly around, careful not to contemplate my dishevelled presence amid the boxes for too long. 'You might even find that you like it.'

'I don't want to talk.'

The air conditioner hummed monotonously.

'I put the number of the specialist on the fridge. From everyone I spoke to, he's the best doctor in the city, and if you can get in to see him, it could really help you. You'll need a referral from the GP, but then, you should definitely call him.'

'I've seen too many doctors already.' I patted the foldout bed with my palm, and it cringed. 'I give up.'

'You have to keep trying.' Her eyes closed on a deep sigh. 'Isaiah said that God's ways are higher than man's ways.'

'Stop quoting the Bible at me, and don't try and tell me

that God allowed me to be sick, like it's part of his plan or something. God has nothing to do with this.'

A severe note entered her voice. 'It's scripture.'

'Can we please hold off on all the God-bothering until tomorrow? The flight was hellish enough.'

She turned away with her cashews, steps slow and hard in the hallway. I turned out the light and I lay on my back, paralysed by the brief conversation. A great wave of self-hate and humiliation came over me as I traced the tender memories of my mother having cared for me over the years, of her endless patience and fortitude in the face of life's bullying and uncertainty and confusion. Although it was now worn with age and she was standing at the end of the hall, her face was the same to me as when I was a boy. In the light of that face, I imagined myself running backwards towards my younger self, to a time before the onset of my illness, with my body growing smaller and shrinking to stand inside my childhood.

Take me back to that one afternoon, aged seven, swimming out beyond the seaweed for the first time, out past the cluster of swimmers to a patch of clear blue water. Let me be free again to float in that clear blue. Something of 'me' lives in that place.

Mother, what was it you said to me that day? 'It's all ahead of you, my boy.' You kissed me on the forehead and rubbed sunscreen into my thin little arms. 'Now, now, don't get burnt.'

In the middle of the night, I woke up soaked with sweat. My body felt like a chalk outline. The weather was putting on a show, with the sound of windblown rain washing the sides of the garage. I got up to open the window. A blast of salty air pressed on my tongue. In the low light, I glimpsed what I thought could be my teenage diary wedged between some DVDs and, to my horror, I saw it was. I read a few pages with my phone light and the horror increased. It was exactly as expected: bad poetry about gardens, bodies and schoolgirls whose names were now a mystery. One line compared a poor classmate to a moon covered in honey.

I crept into the house, careful not to wake my mother, and took the diary and a large pair of scissors into the bathroom. Holding the notebook over the toilet bowl, I cut up the pages like a criminal destroying evidence. Oh, the joy of seeing those bad words flushed away. Bad words were a plague on my life. They were always getting me in trouble, especially at the clinic.

'It's *as if* I am invisible.'

'What do you mean?'

'I mean it's *as if* I am trapped in a box.'

'Can you explain it a little more?'

'I'm not sure I can. It's kind of *as if* ...'

There is immense beauty in bad words, obscure words. Poetry loves those words. Poetry loves *as if*. But not the clinic. Under those lights, only the most direct words will do.

Words like 'broken leg' or 'chest pain' or 'bad cough' or 'headache' or 'stiff wrist' or 'earache' or 'I have tinea under my big toe'. Not 'invisible', and not 'dark pain'. The clinic hates those words. They are too poetic for neat diagnostic categories. Leave those words for your teenage diary, leave them to grow dust in your mother's garage. Don't try to make the doctor into an interpreter, because most doctors have an abject fear of interpretation, especially outside established and long-proven case studies. It will raise the doctor's suspicion, and blood pressure, if you challenge their authority.

In every clinic, under the word RECEPTION, there is an invisible plaque that reads:

NO BAD WORDS
NONE SHALL PASS

I flushed the toilet again, just to be sure. Once I was back on the foldout bed, the rain cleared. The air was all heat. Bleary-eyed, I watched *The Sweet Hereafter* on my laptop, a movie set in the Canadian snow. At first I enjoyed the contrast in weather. But in one scene, which the person who recommended the movie hadn't warned me about, a bus of schoolchildren is plunged into a lake of ice. The children drown, no survivors, their screams echoing across the snow. Seeing the children's wet and helpless bodies reinforced my own helplessness. Here I am, impossibly sick, unable to sleep, with no idea what's wrong with me.

———

One thing I'd never really considered was the complex way depersonalisation worked in my brain. Recent developments in neuroscience have revealed an intriguing relationship between different areas of the brain, known as the default mode network (DMN). Think of the DMN like a computer in sleep mode: when your Mac or PC is not processing any immediate tasks, it is in a low-energy state. In the same way, when the brain is at rest and not focused on the outside world, it activates the DMN. This network gears up when we are engaged in self-referential thinking – contemplating ourselves, our past or our future.

Studies have shown that for people with depersonalisation, the DMN's extreme focus on the self can overwhelm other brain networks, making the individual feel cut off from the world. It involves an acute dysfunction in the sensory cortex in the outer layer of the brain, which disrupts how we process information gathered by our senses from the real world. To delve deeper, the low activation of certain brain regions – specifically the middle temporal gyrus, which processes sounds, and the angular gyrus, which processes language and numbers, memory and reasoning – affects how objects and body parts are perceived.

Take, for example, the hand. When I shake your hand, my brain makes sense of the action by recognising it as familiar. The hand has been seen before. It is matched against a picture of a hand stored in the visual-association area of the cortex.

Within the cortex, the parietal lobe, which includes the angular gyrus, is crucial for maintaining a unified sense of one's body. When this area is impaired, as with depersonalisation, the core sense of 'body self' is affected. This can make the patient feel like they are floating, and when this feeling is sustained, the body self is split in two. It's comparable to stroke patients who suffer neurological abnormalities, known

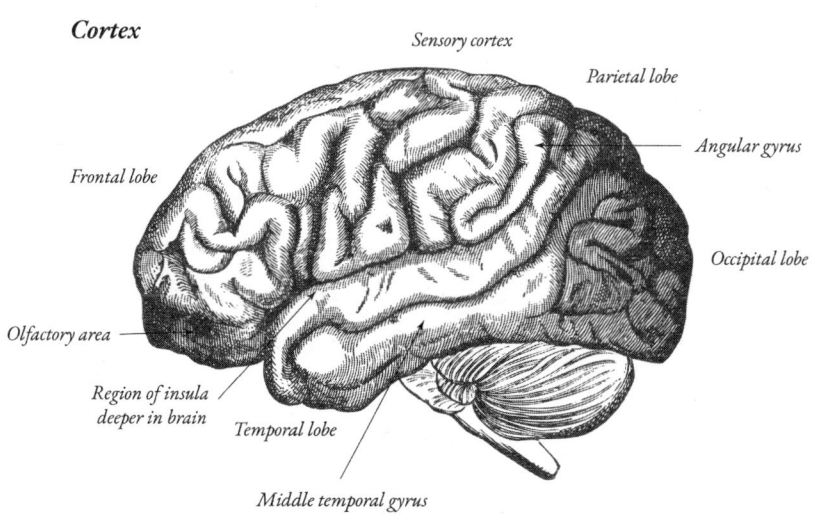

Cortex

Sensory cortex

Parietal lobe

Angular gyrus

Frontal lobe

Occipital lobe

Olfactory area

Region of insula deeper in brain

Temporal lobe

Middle temporal gyrus

as 'neglect syndromes', that make them unable to recognise parts of the body as their own.

Another brain region is also in play. The insula, deeper in the brain, which is responsible for processing internal bodily sensations, plays a crucial role in linking our senses and emotions. It receives sensory information, such as the sight of a rose or the touch of a thorn, and integrates these with an awareness of how we feel: delighted at the rose and repulsed by the thorn. When this function is impaired, emotions become flat. Depersonalised patients speak about the colour of their emotions being diluted, fading from bright colours to grey. What was once joy at seeing the spring flowers is now reduced to the question: Are these flowers even real?

When depersonalisation is the result of trauma, the hippo-campus, part of the limbic system buried beneath the cortex, along with other brain regions, struggles to encode the memory. The limbic system is involved in our emotional and behavioural responses, and the hippocampus plays a crucial role in storing episodic memories, including the time, place and details of events. If you kissed your neighbour, a girl, on Christmas Day in 1990, the hippocampus will remember that it was three in the afternoon, it was Christmas, that she had freckles and long brown hair, and she smelt of fruitcake.

But in a traumatic event – like a mother witnessing her baby being murdered – stress can overwhelm the hippocampus.

Limbic system

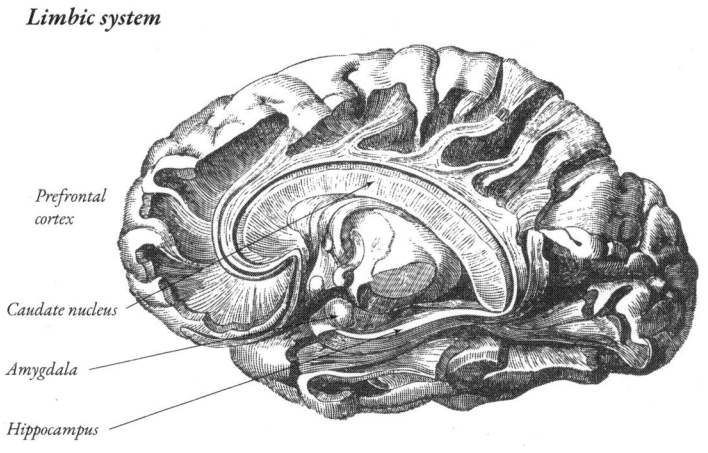

Prefrontal cortex

Caudate nucleus

Amygdala

Hippocampus

The intense emotional shock and high levels of stress hormones disrupt the encoding process. As a result, the time, place and details become fragmented. It's like trying to save a file on a computer while the system is crashing; only part of the information gets saved. If that mother later becomes ill with depersonalisation, she will have difficulty recalling the event because her memory is patchy and disconnected.

———

My brain was subject to process disruptions since the onset of my illness, but it was further challenged when, not long after I arrived in Sydney, an old friend invited me to her wedding. I rented a suit and borrowed some shoes, which were slightly too small. The wedding party was held in a white cottage at the top of a cliff. Sandstone steps ran through gardens of lilies and palms. Guests drank iced water and gin, swatting away mosquitoes in the damp summer heat. Everyone talked about the ocean view. One bridesmaid, already drunk, was barefoot on the lawn, saying how warm it was and how it wouldn't last. A storm was brewing.

At the first drops of rain, I retreated inside to the bar. Wait. Maria? Really? Was that her in the green dress? Her hair was the same, her neck, the way it curved. Oh my God. What was she doing here, drinking wine, making everyone laugh, ordering another glass? I moved towards her, winding through the noise of the crowd. A man was complaining about the review of a charity matinee in the *Sydney Morning Herald*. Before I could reach her, Maria got up and walked towards the exit, past the dessert station and the DJ. I could see the back of her head. She looked agitated. Where was she going? The party just started. I picked up my pace. When I got to the door, she disappeared.

Outside, the storm broke. Rain pelted the roof, pouring from the gutters. The rain was so heavy on the grass it gave off puffs of steam.

A hand came out of nowhere and pulled me outside.

'I saw you looking at me.' It was Maria's voice.

She ran ahead, her green dress trailing on the lawn.

Her silhouette kept shifting, winding further through the gardens, leaves falling around her. The sound of the ocean: *schh-schh*. We sat on a rock. The moss was thick and fleshy. I felt the damp press through my clothes. She kissed me and I closed my eyes at the touch of her lips. Our wet faces pressed together.

'I knew you'd be here,' I said, opening my eyes. 'Somehow, I knew.'

'I almost didn't come. I don't really know anyone.' She traced my jawline with her finger. 'Why were you staring at me?'

'Oh ...'

Her naked face, her teeth. 'You're a cool customer.'

'Maria.'

She squinted. 'What did you say?'

'I love your dress.'

The woman grew puzzled. 'Who's Maria? My name is Francine.'

'I'm sorry, I ... I thought you were someone else.'

She laughed. 'You know, I heard about you. *Chic geek* is how they put it. But I can see you're weirder than that. It's not just the glasses.'

'I don't understand.'

She kissed me twice on the end of my nose, then bit softly into my cheek. 'Don't be so bloody shy.'

I stared at her mouth and tried to wriggle away from her on the rock. Her breath smelt like the brie cheese they were serving at the bar.

'Forget about Maria,' she said, pulling at my collar. 'I'm right here.'

I blinked quickly and teetered, pretending to be drunk. After a minute she gave up on me and began talking about herself, about how much she hated working at the bank, those long hours and horrible bosses, how she never had time for holidays but managed to buy a terrace house in Woollahra by investing in fossil fuels ('There's a lot of cash in betting against climate change'). She planned on buying another investment property because of the proposed rate cuts, maybe in Queensland where the market looked good.

It was almost like I wasn't there.

The storm eased momentarily and she got up, leaving me alone. 'Bye!'

I lay still for a long time, letting the rain drum on my forehead, remembering how Maria's pursed lips looked first thing in the morning, and how, one time, she brought home a thin cardboard box of different perfumes and how every morning, with a fresh scent on her neck, she would ask me to guess what she smelt like, and when I said the same thing, that she smelt like heaven, she would tell me it was jasmine and wood, or fig and wood.

Wet leaves clung to my jacket. I listened to the voices of guests back in the cottage, back in the real world.

I staggered inside and tried to conceal the huge grass stain on my trousers and the mud splattered around my thighs. I was soaked. A large crowd was dancing to Madonna. In the middle, the bride and groom were on people's shoulders, singing and high-fiving, taking swigs of brown liquor from a glass shoe.

'Drink!'

'Drink!'

'Drink!'

Everyone seemed to have chicken in their teeth. Faces began to blur. Noses grew long, chins were raised. Ties were dropped and forgotten. The dance grew faster and tighter, dress shoes on the hard floor. A woman with a peacock tattoo wiped her greasy hand on the hip of her dress and a camera man kept using the flash.

Faces grew other faces, becoming monstrous.

Retreating into the shadows, I was struck numb. I couldn't feel *anything*. Nothing was held within my skin, not a hint of feeling. All I wanted was to stop the flood of pain. I tried hitting my thighs, pinching my face, and scratching my hands so violently that patches of skin flaked off. I dug my fingernails into my ankles, drawing blood. No one noticed or cared. They were too busy dancing. I ran to the bar and asked for a glass

WHEN NOTHING FEELS REAL

of hot water, then hid in the corner behind some plants and poured the water over my hands. My skin swelled up, turning red. I could see it burning. But I couldn't feel the sensation.

Looking helplessly at the dancers, I floated above them, up past the wooden ceiling, past the roof, past the antennas, up up up into the sky.

I stared at the black ocean. Everything was silent.

A waiter handed me some champagne. I was numb when I thanked him and drank the glass. I was numb when a couple pointed at my dirty clothes. I was numb when a box of band-aids was thrust at me. I was numb when I shook the hands of the bridal party and numb when I listened to them talk about their honeymoon ('You can catch crayfish with your bare hands'). I was numb when someone leaned in to tell me the woman in the green dress had gone home early.

The rain refused to stop, growing louder on the roof. Under the eaves, I lit a cigarette and blew smoke at the clouds. I desperately wanted to stop hoping for a cure, to give up completely, to resolve myself to a lifetime of living with this chronic illness, plan for it, expect it, not to be surprised when it erupted in these sudden moments. I felt I had every right to give up. Surely, by now, after three and half years, I was allowed to. Consider the evidence: the pain would not stop or be diluted.

––––

The difficulty of comprehending the strange relationship between my numbness and pain is not surprising when we see the intricate way it plays out in the brain. Our seat of emotional memories, the amygdala, another part of the limbic system, is located in the brain's temporal lobe. It consists of two almond-shaped structures. When we experience an acute sense of fear, during a robbery, say, or in the presence of a violent parent, the amygdala becomes overactive. This often leads to anxiety and panic because the brain is on high alert to danger.

For those of us with depersonalisation, the amygdala responds the opposite way – it is underactive. This is what causes the sense of numbness. Even in situations of heightened emotions, like being fired from a job, where we might expect anxiety, the amygdala does not respond as it normally would. Here, the amygdala is muffled or cushioned, dulling its ability to process emotions effectively.

The part of the brain responsible for registering pain is called the insula, a part of the cortex hidden beneath the groove between the frontal and parietal lobes. When a glass of hot water is poured over a hand, the insula usually responds by becoming overactive – the pain is great. But with depersonalisation, the insula – like the amygdala – is underactive. No matter how much the person tries to increase pain in the body, by pouring more hot water or scratching the skin, if the insula remains dulled, the pain will be diminished.

But what makes it even trickier is, at the same time, the prefrontal cortex, which is located in the brain's frontal lobe and helps regulate the brain's entire network, is overactive. This ensures that the amygdala and the insula, which are already dulled, remain flat. The result is a compound effect of numbness and pain.

We can break this down into a formula for how these brain processes work in depersonalisation:

$$DP = EN + RP = \frac{Amygdala\downarrow + Insula\downarrow}{Prefrontal\ Cortex\uparrow}$$

DP = Depersonalisation

EN = Emotional Numbness

RP = Reduced Pain Perception

Amygdala$\downarrow$ = Underactive Amygdala (numbed emotions)

Insula$\downarrow$ = Underactive Insula (diminished pain response)

Prefrontal Cortex$\uparrow$ = Overactive Prefrontal Cortex (increased suppression)

One fascinating consequence of this interaction between brain processes is the tendency for obsessive thought. When the prefrontal cortex is overactive, although it suppresses the amygdala and insula, which are *already* underactive, it tends to focus thoughts on single objects or experiences. This creates a mental 'groove' where the thoughts get stuck. The process is known as synaptic plasticity, in which neural circuits become stronger with repeated use, much like how a path in the garden deepens with every trip to the shed.

Because the amygdala and insula are underactive, the brain lacks the emotional cues that typically help resolve or shift attention away from these thoughts. The prefrontal cortex is left in a cognitive loop, replaying thoughts over and over, making it difficult to move on.

Take the case of Graham Solomon, a 31-year-old man who was in the supermarket when a stranger walked up and slapped him in the face – a dramatic and unforeseen incident. Graham's emotional response was subdued; he was unable to react in the moment and felt little pain in his body. But he returned home to replay the event obsessively for months afterwards, contemplating the motive, the time of day, the clothing worn by the stranger, and a hundred other things about the incident. Perhaps most crucially of all, he thought obsessively about why his emotions were numb and why he didn't feel the pain of the slap as expected.

Advances in neuroimaging technology have meant researchers can now see how depersonalisation shares a common neurobiological basis with obsessive compulsive disorder (OCD). One study showed that the caudate nucleus, a region deep in the brain that helps control habits and repetitive thoughts, is impaired in both illnesses. With depersonalisation, there is a decrease in blood flow, which contributes to emotional numbness, while in OCD, the region is overactive, making it more difficult for the sufferer to shift gears from one thought to another. The shared dysfunction of the caudate nucleus helps explain why depersonalised patients with symptoms of emotional numbness are also prone to obsessional thought.

Researcher Dr Mary Phillips, working with a team of doctors in the Department of Psychiatry at the University of Cambridge, coined a phrase that sums up how these brain processes work to produce obsessive thought in depersonalised patients: 'thinking without feeling'. With a lack of feeling – emotional numbness – there is a rise in the speed and focus of thinking.

Picture a room with two lights. One is for emotions and one for thoughts. When both lights are on, the room is balanced, just like when emotions and thoughts work together in a healthy brain. But when the emotional light dims, the thought light appears brighter. The balance of the room is now off. Without emotions, thoughts become sharper, harder to ignore and, ultimately, obsessive.

———

My mother asked me to go to the garden centre with her to help pick out some flowers. She said it was a good time for planting. I told her I wasn't interested and had better things to do, but, naturally, I went anyway, wandering aimlessly between clay pots and ferns, thinking how much I hated garden centres.

The air smelt of manure. My mother wore a straw hat and kept picking up saplings, asking for my opinion.

I could only shrug.

'Son, I didn't really ask you here to help me with the garden.' She leaned against a palm and cleared her throat. 'I want to tell you about your grandfather. You know, he's been dead for twenty years now and I miss him every day. I have memories of things he told me ... so many things, so much advice about life. But the one thing he never spoke about was the war, about being out there in the Pacific, in Borneo. There were only a few times when he was getting sick, when we knew it was Alzheimer's, that he talked about the war.'

'What does this have to do with anything?'

My mother lifted her hat, wiped a patch of sweat from her forehead and took a step closer to me, putting one hand in her pocket. 'When I woke up yesterday a story of his came to me. He was in the jungle and he got separated from his platoon and, argh, it was getting dark and he couldn't find his way back to camp, and then he found some railway tracks by the river and thought he'd be okay, but the Japanese were coming and he ran to hide under a railway car. The railway car was blown up and half in the river, and so your grandfather got in the river and held himself up underneath it. All the Japanese soldiers were stationed there by the tracks. They weren't moving, and so your grandfather couldn't move. The strength and the courage he must have needed to make it through that, to hold himself up for all those hours and to survive when the enemy was all around him ... Nathan, you have that strength too. It's in you, in our family, and this thing you're going through, this illness, well, it might seem impossible, but it must have seemed impossible to your grandfather too when he was deep in the jungle. He must have thought he was going to die but, you see, he *didn't* die. He came home from the war to live a long life.'

I sat on a bench next to a copper birdbath that shone in the sun. My mother sat too. She took my hands and put them in her lap. I tried pulling away but she held me close, rubbing her thumb over my skin.

'Do you remember the medal?' I asked.

She narrowed her eyes, and nodded. 'The one that said VICTORY 1945? Yes, you bought it at the market.'

'I lost it ... I didn't mean to, but I lost it.' I lowered my eyes. I couldn't stand to see my pain reflected in her eyes. 'On the day I first got sick it fell into a drain. I tried getting it out but I couldn't reach it. I know it was a small thing, but it helped me in tough times. I used to rub it. The medal connected me to him somehow, comforted me. Now it's gone.'

'It's just a —'

'No, it wasn't just a coin.' I stood up and turned my back. 'It meant something real.'

A man with a wheelbarrow trundled by.

We drove home in silence and I shut my eyes, transported back to my London flat. Reeling from the mirror, I dropped the medal, clawing at the drain all over again, reaching in so hard that my elbow was ready to break. VICTORY 1945. I imagined the medal lying deep underground, caught in a pipe somewhere, and thought, maybe one day, many decades from now, someone would bulldoze the street and pick it out of the rubble.

Later that afternoon, I was in the garage when my mother came in holding a brown parcel. She clung to it, not wanting to let go. Her eyes shifted to the boxes, unable to look at me.

'Is everything okay?'

She put the parcel on my pillow, and said, 'I think today is the right day to give you this.'

'What is it?'

'A memoir.' Her shoulders dropped in relief, and she stood perfectly still. 'When you were talking about losing the medal I thought you should read it, finally. Your grand-father wrote it. He only published one copy for the family.

I never gave it to you when you were younger because it's ... for adults.'

'I thought you said he hardly spoke about the war?'

'Writing is very different from speaking.' A clot of feeling coarsened in her throat. 'And it's not all about the war. It's about his life and his faith.'

I unwrapped the book: *The Wonderful Ways of God*. Its pages gave off a scent of potpourri, with a spine that was cracked and faded. In the middle, there was a section of photographs. One showed my grandfather when he was about my age. He wore a slouch hat and army fatigues, which were loose and torn in places. His sleeves were rolled up. The caption said 'First Day Back, July 16, 1946'. He stood with the men of his platoon on the wharf at Woolloomooloo. His face was gaunt, his body impossibly thin. He was a broken man, a shell, washed up after a bloody campaign.

And yet that smile, wide and beaming, the war finally behind him, the mortar shells and bombing raids, those pesky jungle insects, all behind him. His eyes were bright, looking ahead, waiting for a glimpse of his family. He was returning to civilian life, to suburbs of wooden houses and corner shops, to rose gardens that would never look as sweet and strange as on that first day back.

On the page opposite this photograph was a passage where he reflected on the Baptism of Jesus, how John the Baptist took

Christ in his hands, placed him underwater and brought him into the sunlight. 'The face of Jesus was wet,' he wrote. 'The face of John was wet.'

My grandfather imagined himself on the banks of the river Jordan. He saw himself standing among the reeds next to Elizabeth, the mother of John; and James the Lesser, one of the apostles. With his own eyes, he watched the baptism of his one and only saviour. 'They stand in the river, which is shallow and muddy. The water is slow-moving.' Christ was shaking water out of his hair. Drops clung to his beard. People who came from towns all along the valley were in awe. They saw that this young man was, in fact, not just a man, but blessed by something divine, some force beyond human life. The people began walking towards the man, the one they called Jesus, and among the crowd was my grandfather, descending the bank, knee-deep in the river, closer now, hands outstretched.

The sun that shone on the head of Christ was the same sun that shone on the head of my grandfather. It was heavenly light.

And a line jumped at me off the page: 'The water cleans the soul. It does not harm.'

I looked up. My mother was gone. I wasn't sure how long I'd been reading. One hour? Two? Light was fading on the windowpane.

I found a note tucked inside the back cover. My mother's handwriting was clear and to the point. 'I know you have been putting off calling the specialist. It's been weeks now. But son – call him! The hope you feel, I know it scares you. I can see it in your face, that you can't take the disappointment, not again. But call him anyway. See what he has to say. Your grandfather will be with you.'

The water cleans the soul. It does not harm.

8

Horse Riding in Tahiti

Of all the waiting rooms I'd been in, this was the only one with copies of serious medical journals. I was used to leafing through *Vogue*, *Vanity Fair* and *Golf Digest*, but *The Lancet* and *British Medical Journal* were an intriguing choice for a clinic above Jed's Barber and Shave. In a single issue of *The Lancet*, I discovered articles on cost-effective malaria medication, Japanese health policy and eyewitness accounts of the 1510 flu pandemic: 'a great deal of clearing of the throat that is viscous, slow, not a little thin, and quite foamy. Following that there being sputum, coughing, and difficulty in breathing ... weakness of the body.' It was a sign that this time things would be different.

There was gel in my hair. I wore trousers, dress shoes and

business socks. My mother said it was impossible to get an appointment with this specialist, and now that I had one, it was important to make it count.

Waiting to hear my name, I wondered if I could ever return to my studies and graduate with a PhD. 'Not everyone is meant for it,' my mother said. Maybe she was right. But something deep within me yearned to be well enough to go back to academic volumes and be immersed in the art and literature of Britain after World War II. I was terrified of having to contend with the drowned soldiers, of contemplating their fate, of being triggered, and yet I was still hungry for the lives of other artists and writers. I wanted to commune with them again, thumb through their notebooks and diaries, hear their voices speak to me through time – drown out my own. Surely, if I could manage that, I could better resolve the burning question of my lost sense of self.

Dr C was a handsome man in his mid-fifties with a strong Australian accent, a prominent mole on his right cheek and a light beard. He wore a pair of close-fitting, well-faded blue jeans. His necktie was loose, his sleeves rolled up. Behind him on the wall, instead of the terrible watercolours and inspirational quotes I was used to, there was a framed print of *The Clinic of Dr Gross* by Thomas Eakins, a painting I knew from a course on art and medicine. The painting settled me. It felt like being in a classroom.

'You don't need to say much,' said Dr C, holding up my medical records with a smile. 'I've read over these in detail and from what I can gather, you've said a lot already. I imagine you're all talked out.'

'It's true, I've seen quite a few doctors.'

He sat up in his chair and scratched the back of his neck. 'I believe I can help you, but I want to clarify something. In the patient report, you describe floating outside your body. In the instances where you float, do you float far away or usually stay in one place?'

'One place.'

'You describe it like being in a box of water.'

'Sometimes, yes.'

'And you suspect this is connected to the night of your onset in London?'

'I do, but knowing that hasn't helped me.'

'It's clear to me you've been misdiagnosed with depression. I'm afraid it's a common occurrence with depersonalisation, which, from reading your file, has convinced me is your true diagnosis.'

Depersonalisation. For the first time ever, I spoke the word out loud.

How had I never heard of it before? Now that it was on my tongue, it seemed so obvious. What I knew as my person was in confinement, outside my body. When I was diagnosed in the past I often reacted with excitement, believing it sig-nalled the end of my suffering, that to have a name meant I would receive the right treatment. But as much as deper-sonalisation sounded correct this time, I withheld judgement and listened.

'In your notes, there's something you describe as the great hand, an external force that, you say, manipulated your body from the outside.' Dr C stood up, drew an outline of my body on a whiteboard, and wrote *SELF*. 'But what you experi-enced was not the arrival of something *beyond* the self, but, actually, came from *within your self*.' His words were clear and illuminating, the kind of ideal doctor Amiel had longed for in his journal. 'Depersonalisation occurs when your thoughts become maladaptive, deceiving you about the nature of reality. When this switch is flipped, you experience severe disassocia-tion, what you call floating.'

The air in the room swelled with my sense of shock and revelation. I started tapping my fingers on my knees. He ignored this and suggested we start with a simple treatment.

He opened a drawer and put several items on the table:

— a hessian tote bag
— a half-empty bottle of water
— a thick, fluffy hand towel.

I was to carry these with me at all times. Every morning, on the hour, my task was to dip my fingers into the water bottle. 'Just for a second or two, and don't shake them off afterwards.' In the afternoons, I was to pour water over the towel and wrap it around my hand. 'It's important that your hand remains wet throughout the day. We need you to build up a tolerance to it. That way, when your thoughts return to the night of your onset, of being in the pond, it will become less distressing to live with these thoughts over time.' He walked to the window and pulled on the blinds, keeping the sun off his desk. 'You will become accustomed to being in contact with the element that provokes some of your symptoms, and gradually, the thoughts will have less of a hold over you. When you're driving and you see the ocean out the window, or pass by a swimming pool, it won't be a trigger in the same way because your skin is already wet.'

I felt a tremor in my balance. 'Does this approach work?'

'If you stick with it, despite the obvious distress, many patients find it reduces their symptoms by a factor of ten.' He gave me a half-nod. 'The treatment is called exposure and response prevention, or ERP. It's commonly used to treat people with OCD, particularly patients with a fear of contamination. Say a patient is triggered by dirt, or human waste, the task is to carry a small piece of it around with them. Often the patient will fold a piece of dirt or excrement inside a tissue and keep it in their pocket. The closer to the skin the better.'

My voice grew high and thin. 'Do I have to start today? Or tomorrow?'

'ASAP. But if you need to, give yourself a couple of days.'

He handed me a booklet about ERP, full of diagrams and case studies. The print was tiny and dense. There were quotes everywhere. One scholar said, 'Introducing variability into exposure makes short-term learning more difficult, but enhances long-term retention.'

I understood this to mean that combining the tasks of finger-dipping and cloth-wrapping might be harder than doing just one, but could ultimately lead to a more robust and lasting cure.

But what about medication?

'Let's see how you go with the water exposure before we think about a change in meds,' said Dr C. 'For depersonalisation, the studies vary. Some show that neither antidepressants nor antipsychotics are very effective in reducing symptoms. But in some cases, *combining* anti-depressants with other drugs can help. Naloxone, which is used to reverse opioid overdoses, is one, and the other is lamotrigine, which we prescribe for epilepsy and bipolar disorder. If it comes to that, we'll need to experiment and see how your body reacts.'

'I just want to be able to look at the world in an orderly way. I want to know that it's real.'

'Don't fixate on the idea of order. It will show itself in time, without you trying to find it.'

'How long does the treatment take?'

'I like to say "in good time". Sometimes it can be as little as a few months, sometimes years. Every patient is different.' He popped a breath mint. 'One mantra to keep in mind during treatment is: *You are allowed to cry but not to whine.* Patients find it helpful to acknowledge their distress and get emotional when possible. But to constantly complain about the difficulty of the process, especially to loved ones, can trap you in a negative loop and make you treatment-resistant. We don't want that.'

I took a deep breath.

Outside, the sound of a train, fast and rattling.

———

After leaving Dr C's office, I drove south of the city without a destination in mind. All that mattered was getting away from the garage at my mother's house. I couldn't go back, not yet. The highway thrummed with peak-hour traffic. After an hour, I turned off towards the coast. A sign said I was in the historic town of Helensburgh. Streets snaked beside a creek bed and rows of giant paperbarks. Dirt lanes dropped away from weatherboard houses with picket fences. Sydney was still close, but it felt much further away. I drove slowly, windows down, taking in the quiet.

Two joggers passed one another. 'Are you going to the game?'

On the edge of town, a sports ground was lit with floodlights. A rugby match was in progress, the Helensburgh Juniors vs some out-of-towners. Two enthusiastic mothers held up a makeshift scoreboard that said the Juniors were up by six. I parked the car and walked up a steep incline until I was overlooking the field. Suddenly, it was dark. The grass glowed. Kids ran around like mad things, crashing into one another with abandon. Solid tackles, loose tackles, missed tackles. Scrums barely held together. When one skinny player on the wing intercepted the ball and charged off, tearing up the grass, the parents on the sidelines started shouting like it was an Olympic final.

At half-time, the kids ate oranges out of old ice-cream containers while 'April Sun in Cuba' played over the speaker system. A few image-conscious parents took too many pictures, always with a flash, which annoyed the hell out of the parents who were more chill. Then, the whistle again, and the kids got back out there, dashing and falling under the lights.

Watching at a distance, alone, led me to contemplate how far I had come, how I'd waited three and half years for the correct diagnosis – to hear the word *depersonalisation*. I felt like Robinson Crusoe finally seeing the ship come to rescue him – the vessel that would take him off the island. My quest to find a name for my illness was over. The golden word offered hope, something I could hold onto, a railing to guide me on the stairs. With all the joy of the match, I felt a surge of grief for the time lost to misdiagnosis and uncertainty, to my anger at endlessly probing for answers. At the same time, knowing I was depersonalised meant beginning a new fight: learning how to live with it and how to heal. Questions rushed at me: Would I be able to endure this new treatment? Did I have the stamina? Was now the right time to begin? Did I have a choice?

A parent below shouted, 'He's going to make it! Holy shit! There he goes!' and a kid scored right between the posts.

The roar of the crowd filled my ears.

Back in the garage, a box covered in stamps was waiting for me. A care package from Angela. Inside, a paperback copy of Anaïs Nin's *Delta of Venus*, a bag of licorice and a CD. The note said to listen to the music and report back. Canadian folk songs from her childhood; the songs were flush with nostalgia. I couldn't find a CD player but found a few of the tracks online. One was about a winter night by the fire and another about picking wildflowers at dawn. It was obvious why she liked them. They were about her.

Love songs and a book of erotic short stories were gifts I might have expected from a youthful affair, not from someone thirty years my senior. But that was exactly what made our friendship unique: the freedom to indulge each other's wounds and fantasies without judgement. We could share everything without fearing it would break us. From the outside, our bond might have seemed to blur the line between friendship and something more – romance, love, even sex – but to us, it felt entirely natural, as if we'd known each other for decades. We never slept together, never discussed it either, and somehow there was no need.

In many ways, Angela was deeply conventional. A woman who stayed with her abusive husband until his death and then became an heir to oil money. She collected Impressionist art and knew people who thought Margaret Thatcher was a great empath who saved Britain from economic ruin. But there was a part of her that also loved to subvert the norm, even thrived on it. She told stories of stealing £5000 brooches from Harrods, turning off the gas supply for a racist neighbour and, after a lunch given by minor royals – 'horrific' – peeing on the bathroom floor at Windsor Castle.

Although profoundly damaged by her marriage, her grief and her loneliness, she was completely aware of this fact, which gave her what she called 'an edge', a streak of wildness that erupted at unexpected moments. Having been trapped in a long, loveless relationship, she was accustomed to seeking intimacy and affection elsewhere.

Anaïs Nin once wrote of her deep connection to fellow novelist Lawrence Durrell: 'We skipped the ordinary stages of friendship, its gradual development. I felt friendship at one bound, with hardly a need of talk.'

———

Since the late 1990s, specialised clinics and research programs for depersonalisation have been established in the US, Britain and Europe, which means we've learned more about the illness in the past twenty years than in the previous hundred. There are now large patient samples, a robust understanding of clinical features and a new generation of researchers committed to finding better treatment options. The pace of this advance is incredible.

Much of the pioneering work in recent years has come out of London. A team that includes Professor Anthony David, a neuropsychiatrist, and Dr Elaine Hunter, a clinical psychologist, has not only published landmark research on the illness but, in 2019, helped establish a charity, Unreal, that supports patients and engages in activism. David was also instrumental in setting up the first ever depersonalisation clinic in the UK, based at the Maudsley Hospital in south London, which has treated thousands of patients. The irony is that despite this clinic, and research, my case slipped through the cracks of the UK health system, and I had to travel to the other side of the world to get help.

According to *Overcoming Depersonalisation and Feelings of Unreality*, a book David and Hunter co-wrote with psychologists Dawn Baker and Emma Lawrence, cognitive behaviour therapy (CBT) is the most effective first-line treatment. Designed to address the psychological roots of the illness, the Five Systems model of CBT seeks to restore a patient's damaged sense of control. It recognises that the five systems of cognition, emotion, behaviour, physical sensation and environment are interconnected, meaning that a change in one system influences the others.

Say I believe that 'Because of my depersonalisation, I am not a social person.' Over time, this thought solidifies into a fixed belief. When my friend John Hardcross invites me to a party ('I'm going to play Manic Street Preachers all night!') my belief prevents me from accepting the invitation. I stay home and loneliness ensues. This low mood deepens the cycle, reinforcing both the thought and the physical symptoms of my depersonalisation.

But if the belief is modified – 'Sometimes I enjoy going out to see friends' – I introduce flexibility. The shift creates a ripple effect. My actions are no longer centred around my illness. If I go to the party and dance to the Preachers' hit song 'A Design for Life', I will feel less isolated and more in control. If I stay home, the decision feels less driven by rigid thinking, which allows me to feel physically and emotionally better.

The challenge is that undoing a fixed belief requires significant effort and persistence. Patients start by learning how their systems operate, often through a STEBS diary, where they record situations (S), thoughts (T), emotions (E), behaviours (B) and sensations (S). This approach breaks complex problems down into smaller units, revealing patterns. Worksheets also help, as patients rate their numbness, pain, unreality and problematic sensations on a scale of 0 to 100 per cent.

In David and Hunter's words, 'You will become your own therapist.'

My first week of trying the water treatment didn't go well, but not for the reasons I anticipated. Wrapping the soggy towel around my hand proved easier than dipping my fingers. The discomfort of full skin coverage was less intense than partial immersion; the wet patches on my fingers were akin to sunburn, itchy and sore. But the physical sensations were diminished by a series of intrusive thoughts. I was accustomed to a degree of negative thinking, but this felt different, far more intense. The thought, 'You will never recover,' echoed so persistently that it was as if someone was scream-ing into my ear. Another scream, at high pitch, was 'You will drown.'

These thoughts made it impossible to function. No appetite and little sleep. So I stopped the treatment, at which point Dr C suggested we try a combination of the ERP with CBT. Once a day, in the garage, I wrapped my hand in the wet cloth and wrote in the diary. Sometimes this was simply writing down the screaming thoughts, over and over – *drown drown drown drown drown drown drown drown*. Whole pages were filled this way. The task was to hear the thoughts and write them out. But they didn't stop. I still heard *drown* at high volume. The comfort was in seeing the words, making them tangible. Dr C said this was key for cognitive reframing. Visualising the thoughts and fears would tame them and, in time, allow me to accept them. If I could do this, he said, they would disappear.

I dreaded the flashbacks. They were different from thoughts – memories coarsened to a point. They came in words, not images. Sitting in the garage or helping my mother lift a box of old tools out of the shed, Maria's words echoed in my mind. I heard one line on repeat. She spoke it in the kitchen after I got home from the hospital: 'I can't see you like this.' Sometimes it's pleasant to have a song stuck in your head, the melody, say, of 'A Design for Life', with its synth-sweet chorus. But when a flashback gets stuck, it ceases to become a flashback and cements in place.

The echo of Maria's voice was a double whammy. Her words not only marked the beginning of my illness but were the moment she began to grow distant from me, backing away, removing her love. She could no longer see me the same way. Her one statement set the end of our relationship in motion. I wanted to erect a line of sandbags in the middle of my skull. Something, anything, to block out the echo.

'You seem to be doing better,' my mother said, appearing at the garage door. She wore her old gardening hat, a faded Sunshine Coast t-shirt and khaki shorts.

'Do I?'

'Maybe you can't see it yet, but I can.' She sat by me on the bed, and saw the memoir tucked under my pillow. 'How much have you read?'

'I ... ah ...'

'It's only me, son. You can talk to me.'

I sat silently, staring at the book's spine.

She touched me lightly on the shoulder and said, 'Let me read you my favourite part.'

'I can't remember the last time you read aloud to me ...'

With a smile and a slight shake of the hand, she began. Her voice was soft and careful, as though underlining sentences as she went. 'Living in the tropics brings certain challenges to the lives of those not accustomed to it. The heat and humidity is oppressive. The thought of death ... of death has become more real than ever before.'

'Which part is this? Is he writing about the war in Borneo?'

She skipped down the page and kept on reading. 'Scripture says that we should look not at the things which are seen, but at the things which are unseen. For the things which are seen are temporal, but the things which are unseen are eternal. That is what matters. Peace is there, in that unbroken calm.'

'Why do you like this part?'

'It's where he says *that unbroken calm*. You don't have to be at war to want that. We all want things to make sense, to have peace.'

I breathed in her voice, my eyes falling on her sneakers. They were sprinkled with grains of dirt, traces of the garden she had brought inside.

———

CBT helped me challenge my thinking and recognise patterns of emotions and behaviour, but it also brought frustration. The chief problem was that it felt rigid. My symptoms were boxed in. The treatment was working, to an extent, but the causal relationship between the five systems seemed forced.

Looking for catch-all emotions like 'sad' or 'down' or 'feeling pretty good' reduced the complexity of my emotional range.

The model was too basic. It didn't capture my experience of holding conflicting emotions at once. Because of my numbness, I often found it difficult to recognise *any* emotions. When I did, they were frequently a blend of happiness and sadness, and I didn't know how to interpret the contradiction. I marked the emotions in my STEBS diary, but I couldn't make sense of how these competing feelings related to my behaviour. My sensations, too, were muddled – numbness and pain, hot and cold, light and heavy, all bundled up. Rather than drawing clear links between the systems, I was left confused about how they functioned.

Dr C suggested we try something new: eye movement desensitisation and reprocessing, or EMDR, a therapy designed to help reintegrate the split self with the body. The treatment requires the patient to follow a machine-led light from left to right, known as bilateral stimulation. Psychologist Francine Shapiro, who developed EMDR in the late 1980s, liked to quote from William Blake's poem 'The Mental Traveller': 'For the Eye altering alters all.' The quote reflects the theory behind EMDR – that mimicking the rapid eye movement in sleep helps process traumatic memories. When successful, the treatment can dissolve the barrier between the real and the unreal. For me, in the moment, the light made it impossible to think about anything else. My mind was completely blank, a welcome relief that bordered on euphoria. When the light moved along the rail, the machine beeped loudly, a sharp little horn, and the sound kept me in the present, anchored me.

I'm highly sensitive to different colours, and on my second and third visits, there was an intriguing change to the machine: the technician could now adjust the colours. Instead of the usual blue, there were yellow, green and orange lights. The yellow light was harsh, and I squinted to avoid it. But with the green and orange, something unexpected happened. I saw flashes of apples and oranges in my mind's eye. Unlike with yellow, my brain immediately transformed these colours into familiar objects. This was restorative. When I left the clinical setting and struggled with symptoms the following day, I stared at colour blocks of green and orange, and it settled me.

I have strong positive associations with apples and oranges, which have been symbols of vitality and nourishment across time. As the Greek poet Hesiod wrote in 700 BC: 'The rich earth bore them its fruit abundantly and unstinting all by itself. They lived off their fields as they pleased, in peace.'

EMDR didn't cure my second-body symptoms, but it gave me a tool to manage them. Using the colour blocks helped ease the intensity of my unreality, allowing my brain to rest. While the treatment worked during the sessions and for a few hours afterwards, the relief was short-lived. It was a band-aid, helpful in the moment, but not a long-term solution for a chronic illness.

In the waiting room before one of my sessions, I talked to another patient with a different treatment experience. She was a girl about twenty years old whose chronic depersonalisation turned her life upside down. 'My situation was that my brain was literally stinging in pain from my DP. I could hardly walk or do anything. I'm only a week into the EMDR but my DP is way down, like 50 per cent down. After a session, I feel like it leaves me achy and tired the next day or two, but it's worth it for what it does. I feel more like a person, more in my body than I can remember feeling, like ever, and more capable of dealing with my usual triggers. There's still more to do, I think, but still, it's actually friggin amazing when I think about all the shit that's happened up to now. It's a beautiful world when you can feel it.'

Returning to the garage, I was envious of this woman's experience, wondering why EMDR didn't offer me sustained relief in the same way. I was ready to take up the water treatment again when my mother brought me a new study, all printed and stapled.

'What do you think?' she asked, peering over my shoulder as I read the first few pages.

'Seems experimental.'

She tapped on the page. 'According to this, it's been around for a year or so now.'

'Okay, but my brain will be stimulated with electrical pulses.'

'I'm showing you this because of the great results. Look!'

'I don't want to be guinea pig. Repetitive transcranial magnetic stimulation. Sounds like something that ends badly.'

'I think we can do this,' she said, giving me a big, long hug. 'The machine looks very innovative, high-tech. I looked up a picture online.' She nodded with a smile, eyebrows raised. 'I've got a gut feeling.'

'You always have a gut feeling,' I said, and we both laughed.

Starting this treatment wasn't cheap, but with Dr C's help, I got access to a clinic that allowed me to pay in instalments. If it was ineffective, I could end the sessions without going bankrupt. During my initial consultation, I was assured that while the treatment is often confused with electro-convulsive therapy (ECT), it is completely different. rTMS, as it is commonly known, doesn't require a general anaes-thetic, electrodes or mouth guard. It is far less invasive. Unlike with ECT, which can cause memory loss, there are no known side effects.

As I sat in a comfortable chair, my head was measured against a general template of the brain. In a process called 'neuro-navigation', the doctor located an area, the dorsolateral prefrontal cortex, and said, 'Don't be nervous, just imagine you're horse riding in Tahiti,' before using a helmet-shaped magnet to apply 1 Hz per second. There were 2400 stimulations in total, and with the delivery of each Hz, there was a loud click. My body was stiff, but with no immediate pain or pressure in my head.

With rTMS, the idea is to target areas of the brain that are impaired because of the illness. In my case, the hope was to reanimate the parietal lobe, which includes the angular gyrus, to regain a unified sense of my body. In the lead-up to treatment, I spoke to other patients at the clinic about their experience. A 41-year-old man in part-time employment as a cashier told me he was 'much more awake and switched on to the world'. Continuing the treatment for thirty sessions,

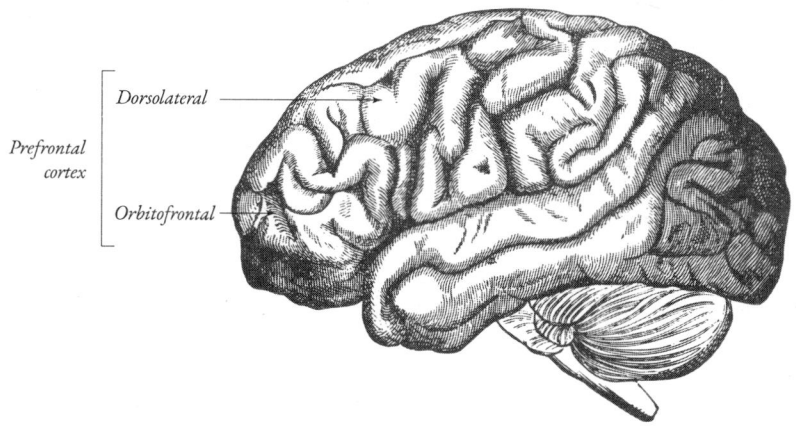

Prefrontal cortex

Prefrontal cortex

Dorsolateral

Orbitofrontal

he reported increased appetite, hearing more clearly and generally being in better spirits.

Another patient, a 29-year-old woman who described herself as 'a long-time tax officer', said: 'After my first session I got frustrated because I thought it wasn't working and I had scalp soreness and headaches. My dreams were weird too, in the beginning, but then as I did three sessions a week I got used to it and the treatment kicked in. My system rebooted and the effect was amazing. I'm so glad I stuck with the whole plan and didn't give up. It got worse before it got better, but the best thing was it *stayed* better.'

I was sceptical about the treatment yielding a similar dramatic improvement in my case, but I found, to my great surprise and relief, that as the sessions progressed my symptoms started to wane. After my sixth session, I recorded a 25 per cent drop in the intensity of my symptoms and at the end of treatment I fluctuated between 35–40 per cent reduction – an astonishing result.

My full treatment plan was tailored to include a combination of rTMS sessions and ERP water therapy. Doing this reduced my symptoms by up to 65 per cent. A chronic illness like depersonalisation doesn't have a clear end point. There is no definitive cure. But the change in me was remarkable. My second-body symptoms were diminished to the point where I regained a sense of embodiment I'd not felt in years.

I no longer perceived myself as completely absent or invisible. I still avoided mirrors, but slowly I grew accustomed to glimpsing my reflection in windows and bottles. These encounters no longer sparked the same panic. My memories, too, became more coherent, forming a clear narrative with a linear time span.

When I mentioned my improved memory to a friend, a scholar specialising in French literature, he said, 'But memories aren't supposed to fit together. Their very nature is incoherence and dislocation. It's all a jumble, which is why they make us feel so strongly – they're always out of sync.' I replied that while that might be true for some, I needed a narrative arc of my life to feel whole, to feel like myself.

I was full of joy at being able to focus again – to read books with ease, do research and watch movies without fatigue weighing on my eyelids. With this renewed energy, I made real progress on my thesis. Even when the words didn't come, my ability to think and reason was much improved. As my numbness eased, the pain also diluted. Days were easier than nights, but overall I coped better. I went for drives, got a haircut, reconnected with friends, discovered new music, bought my mother a thank-you necklace, hiked in the Blue Mountains, and spent Wednesday evenings at life-drawing classes sipping cherry punch mocktails with good people. I was living again, and with it, my sense of self began to return.

One morning – just like that – I declared loudly in the kitchen, 'I'm becoming myself again.' My mother spilt her breakfast cereal, milk dripping from the counter. She took me in her arms and we cried together, then danced to Bing Crosby on the linoleum.

———

'I rang to see how you were feeling.' Angela's voice was bright and generous. 'Did you call that doctor?'

I sat up on the bed, bleary-eyed. The phone woke me from a nap. 'I did.'

'And?'

'I have a new treatment plan and, to be honest, I'm feeling quite a bit better. I've been writing again and yesterday I decided it's time to move back to London.' I looked over at my bags, half-packed, a pair of stripey socks edging out.

'Nathan ...'

'I know, it's huge.' I yawned, and nodded as if she was sitting right by me. 'There's a long way to go, but it's big.'

With Angela's voice crackling over the speaker phone, the garage took on an air of intimacy. 'I thought of you the other day when I was at one of the private galleries. Lisson, I think it was. There was this incredible photograph of people swimming in a motel pool in the 1950s or thereabouts. One girl was wearing one of those old bathing caps and there was just this beautiful atmosphere about it where you could tell everyone was having so much fun, so alive and in tune with each other, splashing and splashing. The photo is black and white and it's by Garry Winogrand, a great photographer. I'll send you the image. It's the kind of art that could make you want to swim again one day. I know water is tough for you, but I think you'll love it.'

She sent the image as a text. On my phone, the photo was dark and full of shadows. The people were swimming at night, under fluorescent lights. She was right. They looked so joyful, playing in high summer. Standing in the middle of the garage, I wondered if my eyes were sharper than usual. The contrast of black and white in the photo looked incredibly clear. I zoomed in, pixels breaking up. I didn't feel any dizziness or rise in my pulse. The water was serene, even inviting.

'Thanks for sending this,' I said, still waiting for my body to have an adverse reaction.

'Now that you're coming back to London, we'll have to make a million plans.'

'Can't wait.'

'No, *I* can't wait.'

'No no no, *I* can't wait.'

'My dear boy,' she said. 'It's been a real pleasure, a really wonderful pleasure.'

Those last words, the emphasis she made on our friendship and connection, have stuck with me over the years. Her comment was about our conversation – a thank-you for the chat – but I've often wondered if somehow she knew what was coming, some light on the stairs she saw and kept to herself, something that told her time was running out.

9

Communion

During my second week back in London, I was at a flower shop in Brixton, dazed among the peonies. Fresh flowers were a bid to make my new flat less dreary. Sun from the windows threw shadows between the stems. A happy couple, proud of their engagement, were taking pictures of bouquets and arguing about the cost of wedding venues. The florist was annoyed. Before I could decide on a bunch, my phone rang.

A man's voice asked if I was Nathan, the close friend of Angela Bass. Then the news: she'd collapsed on an escalator at the Edgware Road tube stop and died in the ambulance on the way to St Mary's. 'A massive stroke.' The man was Angela's son, calling from Canada.

'She never mentioned she had a son.'

'Well ...'

'Angela is a special person.' I couldn't bring myself to say *was*.

'Our relationship was strained. I was closer to my father, and when he passed, my mother and I drifted apart.' His voice was thin and hoarse, a little frightened. 'I think seeing me was too painful for her. I reminded her too much of the man she hated and so she pushed me away. She went on with her life. It was very sad, and it's even sadder now she's gone, but I'm sure she was happier forgetting all about me. Giving up contact – I always hated her for that. I never understood her reasons. At the end of the day, I'm still her son.'

How strange that she never spoke to me about this man, a baby she carried and raised. She was so warm to me, always available, calling me 'dear boy', offering endless encouragement and support, treating me very much like a son. Although our friendship was complicated, because of the sheer gap in our ages, her presence in my life was maternal, a guide to the future.

In the flower shop, time collected – and stopped – at 3.10, refusing to move.

The florist. 'Are you okay, sir?'

Her body would be flown back to Canada, to the prairies she once described as 'small-town quiet mixed with the fire of the Old Testament'. I thought of how much she would hate going back against her will, carried over wheat fields to lie in a church with no stained glass or tapestries. She would loathe the simplicity, the inelegance, the reduction in her finery. All that Protestant austerity was anathema to her.

A memorial service was held in London at a community hall near Bedford Square. Her son, who on the phone referred to himself as 'the engineer', wasn't there. But there were about thirty others: a motley crew of curators, chefs, broadcasters, collectors and one personal trainer. Red tulips lined the podium where people got up to honour her. The speeches were mostly formal and solemn, evoking a world now bereft of Angela's special charm, but the trainer broke the mould with a story of how she once dared him to drink a glass of egg yolks, and when he accepted, he threw up all over her ('She called me rude names after that').

When Angela's favourite song – Edith Piaf's 'Non, je ne regrette rien' – played over the speakers, the magnitude of her loss came over me. I registered the shift, a great ripple in the air, but I couldn't face the full force of my grief. Not yet. I was still in shock.

Angela taught me what it means to share, the way it binds us. We shared everyday details of our lives: the spinach we ate for lunch, strange tube encounters, the delights of the London Zoo, weird tech products, disappointing TV episodes, the problem with ITV news, the orgy of listening to Bach, the orgy of listening to Joni Mitchell.

Sharing my life with Angela helped rebuild my capacity to love. Our friendship was a process of learning from each other and, as St Augustine wrote, 'We learn in order to love.' If the highest and deepest human possibility is the capacity to understand one another, as Augustine believed, then Angela taught me how to understand others better. Knowing her meant that I could look out on the world through her knowledge and experience. She helped me see life differently. First, as she did. Then for myself – anew.

But that was over now. Our ritual of sharing – silent. We shared so much, and so frequently, that I would begin to text her and remember she'd never get the message.

What could I do? I started to commune with her memory. I ate at her favourite chicken spot on Clapham High Street and imagined her presence in the shop, how she rated the kebabs. I heard her voice: 'Too many onions!', 'Better than a trip to Paris', 'Not enough sauce', '10 out of 10'. Sitting at a plastic table, I thought of her mouth taking in the food, it dropping into her stomach, breaking up into her body. Then I took a bite of my own meal – number 4 on the menu, the snack pack – feeling the chicken slide down into my stomach.

Our special proximity.

Walking in Chelsea, I drank her favourite posh lemonade and started to burp. People laughed. I laughed too, then caught myself. Angela would never be able to laugh at me again.

She would never put on a stern face and scold me for bad manners before launching into a burp herself. Angela loved burps. She was so well dressed people never saw it coming. She once said that burping in a quiet restaurant is like punk rock, as if the Sex Pistol Johnny Rotten himself walked in and started singing 'Holidays in the Sun'.

This communion with Angela was vital to my wellbeing. Being able to remember her, the places we went, conversations we had, kept me in touch with reality.

Inevitably, though, as the weeks passed, the strength of the communion began to fade. I couldn't feel her presence with the same intensity. Memories started to slip, becoming muddled and vague. I tried to hold onto these by writing them out in a notebook, recalling whole afternoons, moment by moment. But the exercise only reinforced how much I was losing her. She was fading too fast, and I couldn't do anything to stop it.

One evening I sat outside her house in Bedford Square and the grief finally hit me. It was the recognition that I could wait forever, and yet she was never coming home. Among my tears, a part of me envied her. She knew the answers to all my questions. What is it like to feel no pain and to have no anticipation of pain? What is it like to be free of your body? What of paradise? Now that you know silence, is there peace?

With this grief came a relapse of my depersonalisation symptoms. Trying to hold onto the memory of Angela's body caused a disturbance in my own. My second-body symptoms were fierce, 10/10, overwhelming my ability to function. All the progress I'd made, the work I put in with Dr C and my treatment plan, seemed to vanish in a single day. CBT and ERP were insufficient tools for navigating this kind of obstacle. They were not robust enough. The grief wasn't tied to my onset and the loss of my self, but the loss of someone else's body, and with it, her life.

Just as sharing my days with Angela increased my capacity for love, her death opened me to an even deeper experience of loss. I once believed that the loss of my self took me to the limits of what I could bear. But in grieving Angela, I found that my capacity for loss was far greater than I'd understood. I was in new territory, beyond all recognisable limits, where the healing I had worked so hard for began to unravel.

———

In his book *The Varieties of Religious Experience*, philosopher and psychologist William James relates the story of a teenager who becomes depersonalised in the wake of grief. 'The first time that I perceived that I was two was at the death of my brother Henri, when my father cried out so dramatically,

"He is dead, he is dead!" While my first self wept, my second self thought, "How truly given was that cry" ... This horrible duality has often given me matter for reflection. Oh, this terrible second me ... how it sees into things.'

Sudden grief can sometimes create an obstacle to reality. The shock is so great that the world feels unreal without the person we lost. For some people, like the teenager mourning his brother, this can trigger depersonalisation, and for patients in treatment, like myself, it can cause a relapse.

Grief was a new obstacle for my split sense of self. My second self – the outside observer – looked back at my first self and struggled to reintegrate. There was something in the way. Something that felt *physical*. Patients often describe this mental obstacle in visual terms that feel solid or impassable: 'a brick wall', 'a fence', 'a piece of concrete', 'frosted glass'. The obstacle can also be specific to the person who died: 'his favourite shirt', 'her cake tin', 'a pair of running shoes', 'her desk chair'.

For me, the obstacle was a circle. A fuzzy, pulsating circle. In the weeks after Angela died, the circle changed from grey to a deep black – the end of the colour chart. I was puzzled over what the circle meant, and why it felt so immovable, until Dr C spoke the obvious: 'It's a black hole. A symbol of her absence.'

I had to press through it somehow.

At certain times of day, often mid-morning or afternoon, I tried to help my second self find its way back to my body, guiding it along a mental path towards my skin. I referred to these attempts to reconnect as *flights* (not to be confused with the fight-or-flight response). But each attempt seemed only to strengthen the black hole, as though it fed on my repeated efforts, growing more powerful. With every encounter, I felt increasingly detached.

Which aspect of grief caused this obstacle – this black hole – to grow? It wasn't loneliness but something deeper, what psychologists call 'social loss'. This term reflects the idea that humans draw identity, support and wellbeing from their social connections, and when grief disrupts these bonds, it leaves a distressing void. With Angela gone, I lost her knowledge and experience, feeling myself slowly drawn back into the narrow lens I used before her. She taught me to see the world differently and, without her, I was reduced to that smaller version of myself, forgetting the wisdom I gained between her walls in Bedford Square – a lapse into my prior limitations.

All the places we went and conversations we had were finite. No more. There was such depth in her presence, and she brought such colour to my life, that I struggled to grasp that we would have no more days together. Her charm was unmistakable: the way she railed against pashmina scarves while choosing which one to buy, or how she rubbed coffee grounds into new shoes to make them look worn in. That force of personality had reached its end.

I could only try to bottle these memories, preserve them. But how could I ensure they stayed vivid, that I wouldn't forget or twist them over time? We'd been so at ease together, so free, so unguarded, and now that I knew how precious our time was, I felt an immense pressure to keep her memory close. I wished I could call her, ask how to do it right, how to preserve her exactly as she was. If I were the one to die, how would she have kept my memory alive? But I couldn't call, and she couldn't answer. I was alone in this.

One patient, a 34-year-old woman who worked as a paralegal, told me how she relapsed after the death of her husband: 'I thought to myself, "How is this the same house, the same street, the same car? How is the gate to our kid's school the same gate? It can't be. My husband is what made those things real. He anchored them in the world. After we buried him, and I watched him go down in the coffin, I started to question if I was real too. Maybe I died with him and I didn't know it."'

In the wake of my grief, I couldn't go back to rTMS for treatment because in London it was still being tested in research settings and not accessible through the NHS. Even if I could have afforded private rTMS treatment in the UK, I was not aware of any public access at the time. Instead, Dr C changed my medication to include venlafaxine, along with a new vitamin regimen and magnesium soap. But the anti-anxiety properties of the cocktail weren't sufficient to reduce my sorrow and let me sleep, so I was also given Valium. I started taking this often, as much as four to six times a day, which helped reduce my anxiety levels to a baseline where I could function. But this wasn't a long-term solution, and I knew it.

The main goal was to finish my PhD. Most mornings I woke up wondering if I was well enough to work. Often I wasn't, but I had a decent schedule and did my best to stick to it. To help with this, Dr C suggested I try 'a time-honoured treatment', meaning the approach was antiquated and now controversial. I didn't hesitate. After waking on an empty stomach, I took timed showers – five minutes of extreme heat, followed by five minutes of cold. I repeated this cycle for half an hour, and while under the tap, I played classical music from a little speaker set up on the dirty clothes basket. Dr C said it was important that the music had no voices or lyrics to distract the mind.

On alternate days, I put on Berlioz's *Symphonie Fantastique*, a piece with a few dramatic moments yet otherwise sedate, and Handel's *Water Music*, which, although a bit on the nose, was meant to take the fear out of bathing with its vibrant blend of horns and trumpets and strings. I came to prefer the lesser bombast of the Berlioz. Combining the blasts of water with the music helped short-circuit any looping negative thoughts. I wasn't capable of thinking about Angela. When I tried, my mind encountered either the sensation of the water (even if sometimes this registered as dull) or the music, which was constantly changing.

To finish writing my thesis, I couldn't avoid the drowned soldiers, who raised their wet heads between paragraph breaks or at the ends of ellipses, flashed their wet arms in the footnotes and even, at times, attempted to climb onto the life rafts of em dashes. I cursed them, deleted them and put my computer to sleep, only to boot up the next day to find their cries more insistent.

'Will you tell my wife that I —'

'My life wasn't supposed to be like this.'

'Who the fuck is John Latham? You call that art?'

'There's one pub in Lübeck where I danced as a schoolboy.'

'I only ever swam in the lake at Bodensee.'

'I'm only twenty-two.'

'Angela is never coming back.'

'I'm only twenty-one.'

'The British weren't meant to fight, at least not like this.'

'Maria hates you, every morsel of you.'

'Who will feed my dog?'

'There is no writing down here, under the hull. No oxygen either.'

In the end, I gave up on the screen and wrote by hand, finding that a pencil worked best. Sharpening the point to as thin as possible allowed me to keep the text small, bunched up on the page, and prevented too many gaps. This way, I wrote faster and with greater clarity of thought. Typing it up later proved a challenge, but at the time it was the best way to get the words down.

On the morning of my final exam – the PhD defence – I stood at the back window of the flat, cold coffee in hand, postponing my short walk to the bus stop for another few minutes. The fear was that I might, in the end, have not done enough, have said very little, that my intermittent time in the library was squandered, my debates with colleagues a waste of breath. But after a three-hour conversation in a room above Endsleigh Street in Bloomsbury, it was all over. Somehow, I passed. My supervisor lifted me off the ground in a one-time-only hug and gave me a solemn British nod.

'You have arrived,' he said.

———

For two weeks a year, in the second half of July, London casts a spell. It's an enchanted season, so fleeting that every day of unbroken sunshine feels full of possibility, as if a chance meeting on the South Bank or a Peckham rooftop might change the course of a life. If things are going well for you, with a career on the up, decent housing and an *okay* GP, then it feels like you can rise up with the buildings and accomplish anything. You can embody the ambition of the architecture: ascend above the domes of Westminster and St Paul's, the antennas of BT Tower, the terracotta of the Victoria and Albert Museum, the chimney of Tate Modern, the turrets of the Horniman, the glass of the Gherkin, the needlepoints of Southwark Cathedral.

Inside this spell, my grief for Angela softened, allowing me a reprieve. I felt invigorated, at one with the grandeur of the city, its great promise. I was genuinely happy in a way I had not felt since moving to England a decade earlier.

On the street outside my flat, a construction worker started to sing. The melody sounded like 'Goodnight, Irene'. As I passed him by, he said, 'I never sing,' and we smiled at each other.

Every morning, as I walked around Kensington Gardens, I stopped to watch the light collect around the spire of St Mary Abbots. I squinted up through the trees, keeping still. As the light changed, the cross beamed, disappeared, and beamed again. This quiet spectacle suggested there was a place for me in this great metropolis. The cross drew me in, lifted me, a rootless striver from half a world away, as if the city claimed me, whispering that I belonged.

I found myself in Russell Square, revelling in the fact that my studies were finally over. I was free to do anything: hike to John O'Groats, build a four-poster bed, trawl online listings of exotic bark collections, flee the city on the Eurostar to spend days at Disneyland Paris getting drunk in a Mickey Mouse hat. With my thesis deadline behind me, the possibilities seemed endless, no matter how wacky or impractical.

Strolling through the buzz of tourists and students, I came to a sunny patch on the path and stood turning in place, holding my face up to the health-giving sun. I ran my hand through the fountain and lifted my wet fingers to dampen my cheeks.

And then she appeared – Maria – right in front of me. A chance encounter. Her body blocked the sun. I blinked. She came closer, a crisp baseball cap pulled down over her hair. She wore a sheer white top and a pleated skirt. But she wasn't alone. The man was forbidding and tall, strapped with a leather satchel. Seeing Maria's face after so long was like being blown onto the tracks of an oncoming train.

'What are you doing here?' she asked, sweetly and with genuine surprise.

'I'm just standing here.'

Despite the heat of the day, she seemed untouched by it, as if she'd been able to bottle the crispness of her morning shower all the way from Hackney or Belsize Park. 'There's no need to be awkward.'

'I'm fine,' I said, still in shock.

'You look well.' She turned on me with bright eyes. 'Are you *better*?'

I was never going to talk to her about my health, not out here in the sunlight, not ever.

The man said, 'Oh, *you're* Nathan,' and took Maria's hand, pulling her close.

I tried to ignore him, but he locked eyes with me and introduced himself as 'Maria's boyfriend, the novelist'. Not *a* novelist, but *the* novelist. He was handsome, but in a hollow way that is sooner or later disappointing. To prove he could read, he began talking about F. Scott Fitzgerald's *Tender Is the Night*. 'Isn't it great when Dick and Nicole go for a haircut? Dick has no idea what's about to happen. It's like Fitzgerald is showing us that in the face of Dick's weakness, Nicole finds her freedom.'

'Uh huh.'

'What do you think about that scene?'

I turned to Maria; the scar across the bridge of her nose still there, pressing at a chamber in my memory, the space in the dark where we would lie together and I would stroke her scar, how she would whisper in my ear about our future. Now, I felt that if I tried to reach for her face I might end up in a police station, or at least get into some ridiculous punch-off with the idiot.

With all the politeness I could muster, I asked if I could speak to Maria alone for a few minutes.

'Certainly not,' said the man. But Maria placed a tender hand on his shoulder and said, 'It's okay,' at which point he sauntered off and pretended to look at the flowerbeds.

'Did you ever find out what was wrong with you?' she asked, without hesitation.

'Do we have to talk about that?'

'You were so sick.'

The scent of her fragrance hung in the air.

'You're still wearing the same shoes,' I said, trying to change the topic.

'They're not the same ones.'

'They're the same brand, same colour.'

'I'm very happy with Sammy,' she said, her mouth narrowing into a tight line. 'We're going to have a baby.'

I shrugged helplessly, then flashed an apologetic smile. 'What do you want me to say?'

'That you're happy for me.'

'I ... I ... don't know ...'

She let out a low angry snarl, then took off her shoes and placed them carefully, side by side on the path. 'There,' she said, without looking me in the eye. 'These are for you – a gift.'

She turned away and muttered something under her breath.

I lurched helplessly about in my skin and called after her. But just like our initial break-up, my words came to nothing. She walked barefoot out of the park, hand in hand with the novelist, and as I watched her get into a taxi, I felt the piercing absence of her face, a face that had once loved me, a face that had been there at the beginning of my illness.

'You will drown,' a voice said. 'Drown drown drown.'

It was devastating, crossing back to a place of deep pain and helplessness. Back in my flat, I told myself, 'I'm not me.' My symptoms became the worst since my onset. The dark pain consumed me, as if I'd made no progress at all in the years since she left. I couldn't stop shaking. My vision was blurry, full of dots and specks. I got up to drink water from the tap and felt my second self dragging behind. I looked back, trying to see this sensation in physical form, but there was only the empty kitchen.

The city, which days before had lifted me up, now struck me down, buildings towering over me, ready to crush me, diminish me, belittle me, block out my vision, my dreams, my sense of wonder, my belief in the future. All the tiles, the cladding, the aluminium, teetered on the edge of a fall. It could happen at any moment and I would be flattened, forgotten, pressed underground into the far reaches of a tube tunnel, where, surrounded by a horde of rats, I would be run over by a train pulling into Aldgate East.

The shock and grief of Angela's death came rushing back, magnified by this chance encounter. My sorrow at the loss of my friend became entangled with the heartbreak of losing Maria. She was in a relationship with someone else – someone I didn't understand. How was this possible? How could she have a baby with this guy? I wanted to call Angela and talk it over. But I couldn't. The dreams I had for my life were robbed, trampled on, ridiculed, and what's more, the culprit had terrible eyebrows and a fake accent. But despite his parodic manner and arch douchiness, maybe it wasn't his fault.

A bitter truth took hold: maybe it was mine.

During my recovery, I'd sensed that the loss of Maria was finally receding into the background, but meeting her again was a painful reminder that I hadn't fully accepted it was over between us. I might have buried the loss, wedged it under a rock in my mind. But I never truly faced it.

On a busy corner in Soho, I stopped. It was after ten on a Saturday night. The air was electric with the sound of outdoor diners, sports fans, Groucho Club members and the homeless. Things were kicking off. 'I was on this street with Maria,' I told myself. 'We kissed up against the bricks. I was on this street with Angela. We drank red wine and she told me that stupid joke about George Bush's lobotomy. But now —'

Somebody said, 'Where are you?'

The silence, heavy and thick, a presence.

Somebody said, 'Where are you now?'

I can't remember how I made it onto the bus, and if I really did draw crude faces in the margins of the free newspaper, or if the man in the Sinn Féin shirt really was standing over me with his hand on my shoulder, or if the driver really did slow down especially for me as I got off and walked into Emergency at University College Hospital, telling a nurse I was about to die.

After my successful treatment plan, and my recovery, how did I end up back in the grip of the great hand? How was I, once again, under the cold lights of the hospital?

———

With depersonalisation, relapse, as I found, is unfortunately very common. After the initial onset, there's no clear path to recovery, and even when recovery occurs, it rarely feels complete. Without effective treatment options, those of us with the illness often have a partial recovery before relapsing. The illness remains present, and we must carry its trace. Learning to coexist with its turbulent and unpredictable weather is the challenge. There may be moments of clarity when the world feels in focus again, finally real, only for the great hand to return with new intensity. For some patients, this clarity can last for days, months or even years before a relapse. And yet, despite these periods of calm, it is a brutal cycle. You trust that the world is real again only to have it called into question once more.

In my experience, relapse is almost part of the illness itself, one of its final key stages. This might sound counterintuitive, but the very nature of the illness, with its oscillating symptoms, shifting pains and questioning of reality, means that it can be extremely difficult to realise you're in freefall until it's too late. Despite the severity of the symptoms, there is often a delayed reaction. The question arises: is this descent into hell really happening to *me*?

According to the data we currently have, it's difficult to measure rates of complete recovery. I know, firsthand, from my experience with the community of sufferers, that many people do fully recover, and we should never underestimate this. But as yet, no study accurately reports the rates. In the future, my hope is for a long-term study where researchers follow a cohort of patients over several decades. Such a study could reveal patterns and triggers that the extant research has missed. It could uncover new avenues for treatment – the development of new pharmaceutical drugs specific to depersonalisation, and drug-free approaches that break up the rigidity I found in the Five Systems model of CBT.

To move in the direction of better data, we need to tackle under-reporting. Many of us living with the illness never get a formal diagnosis, making the rate of 2 per cent in the population a conservative number. Misdiagnosis as depression is a major reason the figure remains low, but it's surprising to learn that despite the severity of symptoms, many people choose not to seek help, making it a largely invisible illness. Many are reluctant to pursue treatment, as I was, and even those who make it to the clinic often end up being officially misdiagnosed. A common occurrence is that a doctor will report the patient's symptoms within the larger category of depression, obscuring the onset of depersonalisation, and thus the overall health record. And although it's hard to believe, the medical surveillance and notification systems are not efficiently set up to record depersonalisation as an illness in its own right, leading to more inaccuracies.

One way to approach under-reporting is to look at models for other lesser-known illnesses. With Lyme disease, for example, the Centers for Disease Control and Prevention (CDC) in the US receives reports of about 30,000 cases each year. But the real figure, according to the CDC, is closer to 300,000 – ten times the official record. To remedy this discrepancy, researchers from Columbia University and RTI International have recently developed a data model that identifies areas of the US where cases of the disease go unreported. If we could use a similar model for depersonalisation to identify vulnerable groups, such as adolescents and university students, it could help adjust the 2 per cent figure to allow for under-reporting.

One prediction is that when we see the real numbers, the figure will likely jump to 3–4 per cent of the population who suffer from the illness. That's a staggering 12.8 million people in the US, 2.6 million in Britain, and would extrapolate to about 1 million in Australia. If we can unearth the true scale of depersonalisation, it would not just be an academic exercise, but would force governments and the healthcare system to take the illness seriously. Resources would be allocated, research funded and, most importantly, there would be a shift in how doctors are trained to identify and treat the illness. We need to change the conversation from one of limited engagement and indifference, to one of urgent need.

With a focus on statistics, especially variable and contested ones, it's easy to forget about the individual. But I know that living inside the graphs, columns and spreadsheets, are my story and the stories of so many others. That figure of 3–4 per cent might sound abstract, a scale that is hard to comprehend, but that's 12.8 million Americans who are disconnected from reality, their sense of self in question. These are not just numbers. They are teachers, students, parents, friends. People like me whose pain is still largely invisible to the world around them.

———

Healing after relapse can seem impossible. The slow, painstaking journey, compounded by shattered confidence at being ill again, becomes a grind that feels like Groundhog Day. A friend once described it as 'the most horrific and consequential game of snakes and ladders'. On Thursday morning you wake up with a strong belief in your treatment plan, ready for anything, convinced you're on the mend, only to find that by lunchtime on Friday, you are flush with dark pain, the ladder has collapsed, and all you can hear is the hiss of disbelief, doubt and weakness. All is fatal, or so it seems. These snake-like dips during recovery are what makes the process so long. The inconsistency of your symptoms exacts a cost on the days when you feel slightly better. Bad days leave a trace, making for in-between days, where the struggle lies in the knowledge that more trouble is bound to come.

My greatest challenge was recognising the different parts of my life that were holding me back, keeping me ill. It was a process of compartmentalisation. During a Skype session with Dr C, I drew large circles on an A3 sheet of paper, each labelled with what I saw as the greatest obstacles in my life. I expected at least a dozen – my life felt consumed by obstacles. But in the end, only three circles took shape: my grief for Angela, my heartbreak over Maria, and my depersonalisation symptoms. At first I was sceptical that only three issues could dominate my life with such power. I thought there must be something missing, an unmarked circle hidden beyond the edges of the page. Surely this couldn't be all. But as I sat with the paper, surprise gave way to clarity. I realised it wasn't the number of obstacles that mattered, but their depth and entanglement. The way they fed off each other reinforced my suffering. My aha moment wasn't an epiphany of solutions but of understanding. These three were not the totality of my pain, but they were its engine, and naming them gave me the first inkling as to how I might disarm them.

I pinned the obstacle map next to my bed, where I could see it after waking. It soon became clear that there was a hierarchy of loss within me, and Angela took precedence. I came to see her death as a gift, one that helped me let go of Maria. We rarely think of death as a gift, especially for the bereaved, but in my case it was. At a visceral level, I felt that losing Angela was a far greater loss, that even though we had known each other for a relatively short time, our relationship meant more to me than my time with Maria. Angela had changed me, giving me a sense of freedom, while Maria had trapped me, kept me in place. Angela's passing was hard evidence of my mortality, of how finite my own life was.

When I got an email from Angela's son with a copy of her funeral service in Canada, seeing the dates of her life printed in bold – 1947–2011 – delivered a jolt of recognition, raw and undeniable. Knowing I would die, like Angela, that I would live only a mere pocket of time, was a liberating force that gave me a better sense of my self as whole. Thinking about my death, projecting myself onto it, offered a perspective of my life as linear. As I grew older, I was making my way from one border, my birth, towards another border, the last – my death. Inside this journey, I could be free.

I couldn't waste any more time on the past, on a love that would never be reconstituted or reclaimed. Maria was going to have a family, and a life, without me, and now I, too, would have a life without her. Instead of the great hand, there was another intervention: Angela's voice. She accompanied me on the street, on the tube, to the dry cleaners and the locksmith, and into Sainsbury's for licorice, milk and apples. Over and over, she said, simple and firm: 'Let it be.' I listened to her voice and knew she was right. My heartbreak, which had clung on for years during my illness, finally gave way, and day by day, week after week, month after month, it ebbed away – bathwater that drained so slowly it was almost imperceptible, until, in the end, nothing remained.

As I continued to heal from my relapse, Dr C highlighted my victories: how I adapted well to new approaches in therapy, how I kept up with CBT and ERP despite the treatments' limitations, how I focused on life's minor celebrations, not losses, how my friendships had grown, how I had reined in my perfectionism, how through trial and error I'd reluctantly taken new medications, how we were beginning to dismantle the structure of terror, fear, doubt, alienation and anxiety that accompanied my symptoms and how clarity was returning to my memories. We had reduced the power of the second body. It was fading. As was my obsessive need to free the part of my self in confinement. Instead, I was becoming accustomed to the strangeness of my new self, one that accommodated the part of my self I lost. I had come so far, with so many new tools.

'You are on track,' he said. 'And if the current course of treatment doesn't work, we can always try something new. It's not the dark ages any more. You are not going back to how things were before. Life is different now. Always remember that.'

10

Every Inch of Sand

In the seventeen years since the onset of my illness, I've been through numerous stages of relapse and recovery. As I sit at my desk today, the best description for the state I'm in is that I have partially recovered. Whatever the future holds, there will likely always be a trace of the illness in me. I can't erase time, however much I've tried. One of the hardest things has been accepting this state of partial recovery and resisting the urge we all have for things to be different. During therapy, I've been over my childhood, work, relationships and friendships thousands of times. Every inch of sand feels like it has been sifted through. What I've been searching for is that single, unimpeachable clue to the mystery of why *my* life was derailed and tortured by depersonalisation. But it has only been in recent years that I've been able to accept that I'll never find such a clue, and to try to find peace in the tangled, and sometimes bitter, aftermath.

Acceptance is never really acceptance – it's surrender. When we speak of acceptance in the context of mental illness, it often carries the weight of a battle. We're told to fight for acceptance as if it's something to conquer. Therapeutic models offer ideas like 'true acceptance', 'radical acceptance' or 'commitment to acceptance', framing it as a process we can master step by step, like climbing a ladder. This approach is seductive, suggesting that acceptance is a destination, a quiet garden with birdsong at the gate. But embedded in this notion is a struggle: the demand to fight for acceptance. For the patient drained of energy, this imperative becomes yet another obstacle. When there is no strength to fight, what then?

Whenever I tried to radically accept my illness, my mind's fight for acceptance only increased the strength of my symptoms. Over time, I realised what was truly required: surrender. I hated the idea at first – surrender sounded like defeat, as if I was a German soldier laying down his arms at Lüneburg. But I came to understand that surrender was about letting go of the need for control. It wasn't about giving up or losing my will, but refusing the endless pursuit of acceptance. Fuck acceptance! I didn't want to accept the horror of my illness. Instead, in my surrender – lying down in the fit of the storm – it began to lose its hold over me. Striving for acceptance only fed the illness's power. Surrender, by contrast, drained its fuel.

I've learned to focus on the days when I feel more present, more whole, the moments when I can engage with the world without fear of my second self: the smell of my home library at night, cold milk at the back of my throat, the sound of Art Pepper's saxophone on 'Surf Ride' and 'Cinnamon', walking barefoot over hot concrete, the way Bernini sculptures look different each time. Dr C calls these 'reality moments' and they sustain me. More than that, these moments feel like progress. They are not the grand resolutions I once yearned for, but they are real, and they matter.

Of course, there are days when the loss of my self, and the suffering I've known, feels unbearable. I mourn a life I might have had: deeper relationships, a different career, moving through the world without fear of the great hand. But mourning, I've come to see, is part of living with the illness. It's part of the surrender – the reality of now – not chasing what once was or could have been.

There are things I would like to say to the version of myself who woke up the morning after my onset convinced it was time to die. I see him shuffling about the small kitchen in his flat, the air thick with the smell of oranges and stale coffee, the light low. His steps are hesitant, the simple act of moving over the tiles too strange, too much for the stricken thing he has become. I tell him that even though he doesn't recognise himself, that nothing feels real, not his face, not the teacups, not the peanut butter knife, that his grip on reality will return. His memory is not lost forever.

I warn him that he will be haunted by the space of the clinic, trembling at its white corners, listening for a voice of belief, waiting for a nod of understanding that won't come. I tell him this not to make things worse, but to prepare him, assure him that help will arrive. Not now, not tonight, but it will. There is a doctor and friend he hasn't met yet who will be his essential guide. Together, they will help map the contours of his new selfhood, teach him how to live within its limits.

Most importantly, I tell him to surrender, to hold on. To keep breathing, to mark the breaths, know them, even when it feels pointless. He will not believe it is possible. He will scoff at my words and promises. He will call me a liar, full of empty platitudes. But I'll say it anyway, over and over: surrender.

Over the past few days, I've been going through old boxes and found some things I kept from the time when I was most ill. I have them in front of me now. Faded prescriptions, CDs of playlists I made for sleepless nights, leaves I collected in Whittington Park, and a box of chalk given to me by a naturopath who suggested I reconnect with my childhood self by

drawing on the footpath. There are also quite a few notebooks, which have consumed me the most. They are a record,
however warped and alien, of my thoughts during that time.
On some pages my handwriting is illegible, and on others
it is crisp, full of little poems, quotes and diagrams. What's
missing, and what I'd hoped to find, are any notes I took of
my symptoms. But I compiled most of these in 'The Possibles'
document, which I never recovered.

Just now I've found an old doctor's bill folded into the
back of a notebook. The amount is staggering, and seeing
the doctor's name, I recognise him as one of the many who
dismissed my illness. His office was near the Barbican. Or was
it Crouch Hill? I can't be sure. I have no recollection of getting
the bill, but my best guess is that it was not long after Maria
left me. Oh, that name – Dr U. I can hear his ignorance and
dereliction: 'Nathan, you need to stop wallowing. A young
man like you has his whole life ahead of him. Don't waste
your youth. Believe me, your young years, you'll never get
them back. It's time to get up off the lounge.'

My story of being lost and dismissed inside the clinic is the
story of countless others with depersonalisation, including
the many I've met, or spoken to, in the years since my diagnosis. It's the story of photographers and bartenders, firefighters
and food bloggers, pilots and waitresses, soccer coaches and
art dealers, husbands confined to the house, a hedge fund

manager, a yoga instructor, a Hollywood executive, a piano tuner, and a retired army officer who stopped believing the Iraq War was real despite being told, again and again, that he served on the front lines in Fallujah. One woman collapsed in a KFC car park and became a recluse, sometimes sitting for hours in her wardrobe running a shopping bag up and down her shins. She hoped this everyday object would help her 'walk the tightrope of life'. One martial arts instructor subjected himself to a brutal daily workout, hoping the intense physical contact might alleviate his second-body symptoms. Misdiagnosed, he gained more than twenty kilograms and spent years on ineffective medication. A teenager described feeling trapped in a piece of glass since Seventh Grade, and being told repeatedly by doctors that her condition was nothing but puberty blues. She called it 'the darkest days a person could live'.

When you live with your illness in isolation for so long, discovering a community with shared experiences is a revelation. In this support network, we are bound by not only our symptoms but a shared experience of being unheard, dismissed and misdiagnosed. The capacity for empathy grows once it is shared, and it's remarkable to witness this social body evolve into a league of powerful helpers and confidants. While depersonalisation remains a challenge to articulate, especially to those untouched by mental illness, within this community

I've found the sensitivity and understanding I once thought impossible.

During the writing of this book, which took many years, I suffered a major breakdown, and while at my lowest, in June 2022, this community was there for me, holding me, guiding me out of the dark, helping me hold onto life. I thought, then, that it would be impossible to keep writing. I interpreted the breakdown as a warning not to continue, that the cost of my scribbling was too high, that my poor health simply wouldn't allow it. But several people in the community assured me of this book's worth, and supported me, day and night, through the worst of the hours. Some literally sharpened my pencils, urging me on. Their unwavering devotion and belief in my story, and the need for our collective stories to be heard, is what ultimately gave me the strength to finish.

The activism generated by this network has helped bring the illness out of the shadows in recent years. A historic breakthrough for wider recognition came in March 2019, when Lyn Brown, then Labour MP for West Ham, delivered a passionate speech on depersonalisation in the UK parliament's House of Commons. The milestone was made possible through the advocacy of Jane Charlton, a patient, and Elaine Hunter, a clinical psychologist and leading specialist in depersonalisation.

Addressing the Commons, the Honourable Ms Brown quoted patient testimony. I wept when I heard it. The experience so closely mirrored what I, too, have suffered: 'My perception drew back into my head, almost as though I was now looking at the world from the back of my own eye sockets. I perceived a delay between an external event, and my brain understanding or processing it. Suddenly there was a fracture between the world and me. While my body was still in the world, my mind had become a disengaged observer ... These days I'm in a constant state of grief; I feel as if I'm grieving for my own death, even if I seem to be around to witness it.' Brown also argued for better training of medical professionals and improved services for depersonalised patients in the NHS, and said: 'The invisibility of the illness makes it all the more important that we speak about it in this place.'

Being part of the depersonalisation community also opened me up to the idea, once again, of romantic love – its many possibilities. This transformation unfolded over years, shaped by the guidance of people who helped me confront how the illness complicates relationships. I feared telling would-be partners that depersonalisation robbed me of the ability to love, that I couldn't feel the way they deserved. I didn't want to diminish love but to reclaim it, to understand its unpredictable rhythms and pleasures. Yet who would accept my leaky baggage? Who would help me make love feel real? It seemed an impossible dilemma, but the community offered reassurance: my struggles were far from unique.

Love spares no one, nor should it. The question was whether I could navigate a 'middle ground' of feeling where I and a would-be partner could find comfort in the limited love I could offer. In dating, I came to appreciate the intense growth required to meet so many people of different personalities and ages. Somehow, in the neon glow of a bar, the corner table at Mr Wong's, or a 2 pm picnic that stretched into dusk, I found that the acute consciousness of my illness lifted in their presence. I was able to flirt, joke and speak without hesitation. 'I need you to know I might not be able to love you the way you need. I might not be able to *feel* love how others do.'

The love I sought was alive with beauty and vigour, but I knew vigour might be beyond my reach or, at best, subdued. I believed that relying solely on the beauty of love, without its emotional depth, would leave me unprotected, unable to sustain or renew myself. I was wrong, and the community helped me see this. A fellow patient reassured me that beauty has its own innate vigour, a unique kind of feeling. It took time for me to reconcile myself to the limitations of this feeling, but slowly I began to hope that, one day, I might meet someone with whom I could share my life, and – I dared to hope – have a family.

My youth was behind me. I carried its trouble, the inner scars. Still I yearned for what F. Scott Fitzgerald wrote about his wife Zelda: 'I fell in love with her courage, her sincerity, and her flaming self respect. And it's these things I'd believe in ... I love her and that's the beginning and end of everything.'

I am now married to a philosopher named Laura who likes to steal sips of my coffee, celebrate Christmas in January and buy me Japanese stationery. We met by chance on a small island called Dangar while both of us were contemplating a swim in the Hawkesbury River. Sun poured over the landscape. That day, I was the only one who swam. Laura sat at the end of the jetty, urging me on in the current. Now we have every day together, laughing, cooking and debating at all hours. As I write this, Laura is pregnant with our first child, a baby girl. My great hope is for my daughter to know the love of her mother and father, and for her to experience true freedom in this one blessed life.

Epilogue

The foundation of my new peace and equilibrium began when I returned to the Hampstead pond, the last, excruciating step in a long course of treatment. I never imagined it would be possible to return to that terrifying stretch of water, one that ripped my life from its course and my sense of self from my skin. How is it possible to face such a place again? Would it lead to some new catastrophe, plunge me back into hell?

One afternoon in high summer, I made the trek. Having sold my bicycle years before, when Maria and I broke up, I asked a friend if I could borrow his. It was an old mountain bike with a rusty bell. Setting off, my hands were easy on the handlebars, sweat building on my forehead. The streets were riddled with cars, yet my heart rate was steady. Heads hogged the pavement. As I rode, it was as if the bicycle were resisting the route on my behalf, stuttering in and out of back lanes, over thin green lawns, climbing up and up. Out the front of a butcher's shop, a group of men, fresh from the pub, were singing a song about a prison ship that sailed for Botany Bay. They waved and pointed at me as I passed by, one of them imitating a wobble as if to test my composure.

After locking up the bike, I stood in front of a sign that said WALKWAY, whose ragged letters had been burnt into me since the night of my onset. All I had to do was keep going. Take it slowly. Follow the bitumen. I wondered if my eyes were more alert than usual. The white letters on the sign were incredibly clear as I looked back and forth between the white and the black.

When I reached the top of Hampstead Heath, the midday sun among the oaks had a gorgeous, sensuous clarity. I drifted restlessly among them, fingering their bark, leaning up against them, distracting my nerves by wondering how old they were and if the poet John Keats, whose house was nearby, ever climbed them. Picnickers were strewn over the hillside, smoke rising from portable barbecues, while toddlers dressed in Ralph Lauren tried and failed to fly a kite. Several women, who looked like Roman tourists, were dressed stiffly in tight black dresses and heels, and a very beautiful boy of about thirteen was standing with them, bored, wearing a leather jacket with a green t-shirt beneath.

I followed the smell of sunscreen down to the pond. Although I knew I'd have flashbacks, as I approached the edge they came at me with such incredible force I lost my balance, toppling over onto the grass. I closed my eyes. A pulse rose in my chest and I dug my nails into my palms, scratching and scratching, before retreating up the hill to sit behind a tree, facing away from the water. I pulled a photo of my grandfather out of my pocket and rubbed it along my arms. I carried it everywhere, as I'd done with the VICTORY 1945 medal years before.

Standing up again, I felt the itch of adrenaline spread through me. All I had to do was collect the bicycle and trace the same route home. In my mind's eye, the flat beckoned. I saw my body on the stairs, then easy on the lounge, nothing to answer for. Maybe I'd put on a record, order food, watch a long movie.

But I'd prepared for this in therapy.

I would finish this.

People of all ages were jumping in, crying out, a band of revellers from Jericho. Hip-hop played from a boombox, and lines of sunbathers cosied up on towels. In blue shorts, I made my way along the jetty.

My mother's voice: 'The railway car was blown up and half in the river, and so your grandfather got in the river and held himself up ...'

The pact I made with myself was that no matter what, when I got to the end, there would be no pause. I had to leap straight into the water —

When my head broke the surface moments later, I could taste the water on my tongue and feel the sting of it in my nose. Patches of sunlight sprinkled before me, broken by eager teenagers in the midst of a game. I surrendered to the water and swam out to the middle, letting the water rush over my head and flood my ears. I swam for an hour, floating on my back, blinking at the sky, trying to stay in the present, part of the consciousness of the hour, the minute, the second. When thoughts did come, I was able to parse them with fresh strokes, finding new areas to swim between the moss and the reeds.

Finally, I swam back to the middle.

I was me, and I was going into the afternoon, the late afternoon, the evening, all through the night.

In the morning, too, sunlight or not – me.

Resources

Initiative for Depersonalization Studies (IDS)
    depersonalization.info

Australia
This Way Up
    Clinical Research Unit at St Vincent's Hospital, Sydney
    thiswayup.org.au

United Kingdom
Unreal UK
    unrealcharity.com

The Maudsley Depersonalisation Disorder Service
    slam.nhs.uk/dissociative-disorders

United States
The Sylvia Brafman Mental Health Center
    Specialist depersonalisation treatment
    sylviabrafman.com

Further reading

David, A., et al., *Overcoming Depersonalisation and Feelings of Unreality: A Self-Help Guide Using Cognitive Behavioural Techniques*, London: Robinson, 2007

Endnotes

Interviews conducted by the author are referenced throughout the text and form the basis for quoted material not otherwise attributed to published sources.

Epigraph
v   The book's epigraph is taken from a speech given by David Foster Wallace in March 1998 at a symposium on Franz Kafka, which was sponsored by the PEN American Center in New York City to celebrate a new translation of Kafka's *The Castle* by Schocken Books. An excerpt of the speech, originally titled 'Some Remarks on Kafka's Funniness from Which Probably Not Enough Has Been Removed', appeared in *Harper's Magazine* as 'Laughing with Kafka', July 1998, pp. 23–27.

2: The Possibles
27   'I have no self ...': American Psychiatric Association, *Diagnostic and Statistical Manual of Mental Disorders*, 5th edn, Arlington, VA: American Psychiatric Association, p. 302.
28   'it is estimated that more than 75 million people worldwide suffer from the illness ...': Hunter, E., et al., 'The Epidemiology of Depersonalisation and Derealisation: A Systematic Review', *Social Psychiatry and Psychiatric Epidemiology*, vol. 38, no. 1, 2004, pp. 9–18.

28 'It is as if the real me is taken out and put on a shelf or stored somewhere ...': Simeon, D., et al., 'Feeling Unreal: 30 Cases of DSM-III-R Depersonalization Disorder', *American Journal of Psychiatry*, vol. 154, no. 8, 1997, pp. 1107–13.

28 'It was something like waking up to find that you're in a coffin ...': Simeon, D. & Abugel, J., *Feeling Unreal: Depersonalization Disorder and the Loss of the Self*, Oxford: Oxford University Press, 2006, p. 42.

32 'with the devil to darken the spirit ...': Augustine of Hippo, *The Literal Meaning of Genesis*, vol. 1, trans. Taylor, J.H., New York: Newman Press, 1982, p. 130.

34 'The water is rising. As he's going down, he slips ...': Bennett, A., '29 March 1986', *Diaries 1980–1990*, CD, London: BBC Audio, 2009.

43 'In the general population, 50–70 per cent of people report ...': Hunter, E., et al., 'The Epidemiology of Depersonalisation and Derealisation', pp. 9–18.

46 'Based on data from the National Health Service in the UK ...': Hunter, E., et al., 'Depersonalisation and Derealisation: Assessment and Management', *BMJ: British Medical Journal*, vol. 356, article no. j745, 2017, p. 1.

46 'In the US, depersonalisation is classified as rare ...': National Organization for Rare Disorders, 'Depersonalization Disorder', <rarediseases.org/rare-diseases/depersonalization-disorder>.

47 'The National Institutes of Health (NIH) also defines ...': National Institutes of Health (NIH), 'Rare Diseases', <rarediseases.info.nih.gov/about>.

47 'Recent studies show that depersonalisation affects at *least* 1 per cent ...': Michal, M., et al., 'A Case Series of 223 Patients with Depersonalization-derealization Syndrome', *BMC Psychiatry*, vol. 16, no. 203, 2016, p. 2; Yang, J., et al., 'The Prevalence of Depersonalization-derealization Disorder: A Systematic Review', *Journal of Trauma and Dissociation*, vol. 24, no. 1, article no. 203, 2023, p. 8.

47 'The ICD-11, a medical classification list ...': World Health Organization (WHO), 'ICD-11: International Classification of Diseases 11th Revision', <icd.who.int/en>.

3: Uncomfortably Numb

57   'I sometimes smack my hand or pinch my leg ...': Simeon, D. & Abugel, J., *Feeling Unreal*, p. 16.

59   'I see my hand touching objects ...': Sartre, J.-P., *Being and Nothingness: An Essay on Phenomenological Ontology*, trans. Barnes, H.E., Oxford: Routledge, 2003, p. 328.

59   'I am not solid, but hollow ...': Plath, S., *The Unabridged Journals of Sylvia Plath*, ed. Kukil, K.V., New York: Anchor, 2000, p. 60.

62   'Barber calls it *the pain affect* ...': Barber, T., 'The Effects of "Hypnosis" on Pain: A Critical Review of Experimental and Clinical Findings', *Psychosomatic Medicine*, vol. 25, 1963, p. 304.

67   'Love is like a fever which comes ...': Stendhal, *Love*, trans. The Merlin Press, London: Penguin, 1975, p. 51.

67   'If in the midst of pleasure ...': Stendhal, *Love*, p. 52.

68   'One depersonalisation patient, a 22-year-old postman ...': Ghosh, S., et al., 'A Case Presented with "As If" Phenomenon', *Indian Journal of Psychiatry*, vol. 49, no. 4, 2007, pp. 292–93.

68   'somewhere else and hollow, with nothing but the skin ...': Salgado, A., et al., 'Depersonalisation and Derealisation Syndrome: Report on a Case Study and Pharmacological Management', *Brazilian Journal of Psychiatry*, vol. 34, no. 4, 2012, p. 505.

70   'something new, with a life of its own, its own biology ...': Twilley, N., 'The Neuroscience of Pain', *New Yorker*, 2 July 2018, <www.newyorker.com/magazine/2018/07/02/the-neuroscience-of-pain>.

72   'He felt nothing at all, and heard nothing ...': Yates, R., *Disturbing the Peace*, London: Vintage, 2008, p. 239.

4: The Invisible Baby

81   'If we cannot see ourselves as "I", how can we possibly see the world of creation?': Newman's question is paraphrased from the following text: 'If I looked into a mirror, and did not see my face, I should have the sort of feeling which actually comes upon me, when I look into this living busy world, and see no reflexion of its Creator ...' Newman, J.H., *Apologia Pro Vita Sua*, London: Longmans, Green, and Co., 1902, p. 241.

83 'It is miserable, we think, to be deprived of the light ...': Smith, A., *The Theory of Moral Sentiments*, Cambridge: Cambridge University Press, 2004, p. 16.

88 'as if the content were not going in ...': Krishna, C., et al., 'Depersonalisation-derealisation Syndrome: A Case Report', *Telangana Journal of Psychiatry*, vol. 6, no. 2, 2020, pp. 185–86.

89 'couldn't feel the sensation of food and drink ...': Chee, K.T. & Wong, K.E., 'Depersonalisation Syndrome – A Report of 9 Cases', *Singapore Medical Journal*, vol. 31, no. 4, 1990, pp. 331–34.

89 'According to philosopher Martin Heidegger, the self is defined by ...': Heidegger, M., *Being in Time*, trans. Stambaugh, J., Albany, NY: State University of New York Press, 2010, pp. 112–36.

93 'Evan is not psychotic. He has intact "reality testing" about his depersonalisation ...': Simeon, D. & Abugel, J., *Feeling Unreal*, p. 32.

5: All Is Strange To Me

101 'I find myself regarding existence as though from beyond the tomb ...': Amiel, H.-F., *n's Journal: The Journal Intime of Henri-Frédéric Amiel*, trans. Ward, Mrs H., London: Macmillan, 1921, p. 275.

102 'Why do doctors so often make mistakes? Because they are not ...': Amiel, H.-F., *Amiel's Journal*, p. 207–208.

105 'I will have none of these passions of straw ...': Amie, H.-F.l, *Amiel's Journal*, p. 30.

106 'My soul is dying, my body is dying ...': Amiel, H.-F., *Amiel's Journal*, p. 251.

106 'I am always waiting for the woman ...': Amiel, H.-F., *Amiel's Journal*, p. 56.

107 'I will not go looking for keys ...': Breton, A., *Nadja*, trans. Howard, R., London: Penguin, 1999, p. 18.

108 'Each of my senses, each part of my proper self is ...': Sierra, M., *Depersonalization: A New Look at a Neglected Syndrome*, Cambridge: Cambridge University Press, 2009, p. 8.

109 'automatic acts ...': Dugas, L., trans. Sierra, M., 'A Case of Depersonalization', *History of Psychiatry*, vol. 7, no. 27, 1996, pp. 455–61.

111 'All possibilities are closed ...': Amiel, H.-F., *Amiel's Journal*, p. 216.

111 'in health there is liberty ...': Amiel, H.-F., *Amiel's Journal*, p. 104.

112 'Shorvon concluded that depersonalisation was ...': Shorvon, H., 'A Depersonalisation Syndrome', *Proceedings of the Royal Society of Medicine*, vol. 39, no. 12, 1946, pp. 779–92.

115 'no longer sufficient for researchers ...': Winerman, L., 'NIMH Funding to Shift Away from DSM Categories', *Monitor on Psychology*, vol. 44, no. 7, 2013, p. 10.

6: The Burning Question

123 '*Among the rain and stone places* ...': Larkin, P., 'Climbing the Hill within the Deafening Wind', *The North Ship*, London: Faber & Faber, 1945, p. 11.

126 'Herman challenges the view that ...': Herman, J., *Trauma and Recovery*, New York: Basic Books, 1997, pp. 45–63.

127 'Dr Emma Černis, a clinical psychologist at the University of Birmingham ...': Perkins, J., *Life on Autopilot: A Guide to Living with Depersonalization Disorder*, London: Jessica Kingsley Publishers, 2021, p. 56.

128 'You must respect your stepfather ...': Neacșu, V.C., 'Clinical Inclusion of Dissociative Episodes – A Case Study', *Europe's Journal of Psychology*, vol. 3, no. 2, article no. 399, 2007.

128 'The wasteland limbo in which I currently reside is ...': Barglow, P., 'Numbing after Rape, and Depth of Therapy', *American Journal of Psychotherapy*, vol. 68, no. 1, 2014, pp. 117–39.

130 'I sat down on my bed, and began to sob violently ...': Newman, J.H., *Apologia*, p. 241.

130 'I wish to be known as a living man ...': 'Preface', Newman, *Apologia*, p. xxiv.

132 'Kari Franson, a professor of clinical pharmacy ...': Franson, K., 'Effects of Marijuana Use on Developing Adolescents', ATTC Network, YouTube, 31 March 2015, accessed 14 August 2024, <www.youtube.com/watch?v=nepWLG7RF34>.

132 'In one study at Mount Sinai Hospital ...': Simeon, D., et al., 'Feeling Unreal: A Depersonalization Disorder Update of 117 Cases', *Journal of Clinical Psychiatry*, vol. 64, no. 9, 2003, pp. 990–97.

132 'One eighteen-year-old girl said that after getting sober she was ...':
Unknown, '18-year-old Girl from Ohio with Marijuana-induced
Depersonalization Disorder', Reddit, 31 October 2011,
<www.reddit.com/r/IAmA/comments/lvthl/
iama_18yearold_girl_from_ohio_with/?rdt=43813>.

132 'One seventeen-year-old boy presented to the emergency
department ...': Khalid-Khan, S., et al., 'A Case of Prolonged
Depersonalisation Following Cannabis Use in an Adolescent Male',
Austin Journal of Clinical Case Reports, vol. 3, no. 2, article no. 1088,
2016.

134 'One study found that seven out of forty patients ...': Medford, N.,
et al., 'Chronic Depersonalisation Following Illicit Drug Use: A
Controlled Analysis of 40 Cases', *Addiction*, vol. 98, no. 12, 2003,
pp. 1731–36.

134 'Another found that 97 out of 608 patients ...': Evans, J., et al.,
'Extended Difficulties Following the Use of Psychedelic Drugs:
A Mixed Methods Study', *PLOS One*, vol. 18, no. 10, article no.
e0293349, 2023.

134 'I felt like the person I was before had been ...': Evans, J., et al.,
'Extended Difficulties', p. 16.

136 'This living death, this half-life, is unbearable ...': Kruse, J.A., 'Late
Thoughts: Reconsiderations from the Matratzengruft', in Cook,
R.F. ed., *A Companion to the Works of Heinrich Heine*, London:
Macmillan, 1921, p. 275.

137 'I have a double, another poor wretch that is coupled to me ...':
Heine, H., *Selected Verse*, trans. Branscombe, P., London: Penguin,
2013, pp. 267–68.

137 'I must leave all that made the world so precious ...': Heine, H.,
Selected Verse, pp. 267–68.

138 'I've battled depersonalisation so bad it's not even funny ...':
Unknown, 'Age 21 – Depersonalisation: A 90-day Report', Your
Brain on Porn, 25 September 2013, <www.yourbrainonporn.
com/rebooting-accounts/rebooting-accounts-page-1/
age-21-depersonalization-a-90-day-report>.

139 'During the COVID-19 pandemic, there was an exponential
rise ...': Ciaunica, A., et al., 'Zoomed Out: Digital Media Use and

Depersonalisation Experiences During the COVID-19 Lockdown', *Scientific Reports*, vol. 12, article no. 3888, 2022.

139 'As early as March 2020, worldwide internet use increased ...': Beech, M., 'COVID-19 Pushes up Internet Use 70% and Streaming More than 12%, First Figures Reveal', *Forbes*, 26 March 2020, <www.forbes.com/sites/markbeech/2020/03/25/covid-19-pushes-up-internet-use-70-streaming-more-than-12-first-figures-reveal>.

139 'Zoom usage increased by a factor of ten ...': De, R., et al., 'Impact of Digital Surge During COVID-19 Pandemic: A Viewpoint on Research and Practice', *International Journal of Information Management*, vol. 55, article no. 102171, 2020.

140 'a recent study conducted by the Department of Psychiatry at the University of Bonn ...': Peckmann, C., et al., 'Virtual Reality Induces Symptoms of Depersonalization and Derealization: A Longitudinal Randomized Control Trial', *Computers in Human Behavior*, vol. 131, article no. 107233, 2022.

140 'The feeling of immersion, whether physical or psychological in nature, allows the user ...': Aardema, F., et al., 'Virtual Reality Induces Dissociation and Lowers Sense of Presence in Objective Reality', *Cyberpsychology Behavior and Social Networking*, vol. 13, no. 4, 2010, pp. 429–35.

141 'Current consensus among behavioural scientists indicates that by 2030 ...': Yogesh, D.K., et al., 'Metaverse Beyond the Hype: Multidisciplinary Perspectives on Emerging Challenges, Opportunities, and Agenda for Research, Practice and Policy', *International Journal of Information Management*, vol. 66, article no. 102542, 2022; Ericsson, 2020, 'The Dematerialized Office: A Vision of the Internet of Senses in the 2030 Future Workplace', 2020, <www.ericsson.com/4ab04c/assets/local/reports-papers/industrylab/doc/demateralized-office-report.pdf>.

7: Two Lights

154 'Studies have shown that for people with depersonalisation, the DMN's extreme focus ...': Zheng, S., et al., 'Unraveling the Brain Dynamics of Depersonalization-derealization Disorder: A Dynamic Functional Network Connectivity Analysis', *BMC Psychiatry*,

vol. 24, article no. 685, 2024; Fang, A., et al., 'Maladaptive Self-focused Attention and Default Mode Network Connectivity: A Transdiagnostic Investigation across Social Anxiety and Body Dysmorphic Disorders', *Social Cognitive and Affective Neuroscience*, vol. 17, no. 7, 2022, pp. 645–54.

155 'When this area is impaired, as with depersonalisation …': Simeon, D. & Abugel, J., *Feeling Unreal*, pp. 106–107.

165 'One study showed that the caudate nucleus …': Phillips, M., et al., 'Depersonalization Disorder: A Functional Neuroanatomical Perspective', *Stress* (Amsterdam, Netherlands), vol. 6, no. 3, 2003, pp. 157–65.

166 'thinking without feeling': Phillips, M., et al., 'Depersonalization Disorder: Thinking without Feeling', *Psychiatry Research*, vol. 108, no. 3, 2001, pp. 145–60.

8: Horse Riding in Tahiti

173 'a great deal of clearing of the throat that is viscous …': Morens, D., et al., 'Eyewitness Accounts of the 1510 Influenza Pandemic in Europe', *The Lancet*, vol. 376, no. 9756, 2010, pp. 1894–95.

178 'Introducing variability into exposure …': Text in the booklet paraphrased from Bjork, E.L. & Bjork, R.A., 'Making Things Hard on Yourself, but in a Good Way: Creating Desirable Difficulties to Enhance Learning', in Gernsbacher, M.A. & Pomerantz, J., eds, *Psychology and the Real World: Essays Illustrating Fundamental Contributions to Society*, New York: Worth, 2009, pp. 58–59.

183 'We skipped the ordinary stages of friendship …': Nin, A., *The Diary of Anaïs Nin, Volume Two: 1934–1939*, Boston, MA: Mariner Books, 1970, p. 223.

185 'You will become your own therapist …': David, A., et al., *Overcoming Depersonalisation and Feelings of Unreality*, London: Robinson, 2012, p. 2.

189 'Psychologist Francine Shapiro, who developed EMDR …': Shapiro, F., 'The Role of Eye Movement Desensitization and Reprocessing (EMDR) Therapy in Medicine: Addressing the Psychological and Physical Symptoms Stemming from Adverse Life Experiences', *Permanente Journal*, vol. 18, no. 1, 2014, p. 77.

190 'The rich earth bore them its fruit ...': Hesiod, *The Poems of Hesiod: Theogony, Works and Days, and The Shield of Herakles*, trans. Powell, B.B., Berkeley, CA: University of California Press, 2017, pp. 175–76.

9: Communion

202 'We learn in order to love ...': Hitz, Z., *Lost in Thought: The Hidden Pleasures of an Intellectual Life*, Princeton, NJ: Princeton University Press, 2020, p. 111.

204 'The first time that I perceived that I was two was at ...': James, W., *The Varieties of Religious Experience*, London: Routledge, 2002, p. 133.

206 'social loss ...': Harvey, J.H., et al., 'Toward a Psychology of Loss', *Psychological Science*, vol. 9, no. 6, 1998, pp. 429–34.

219 'researchers from Columbia University and RTI International ...': Bisanzio, D., et al., 'Current and Future Spatiotemporal Patterns of Lyme Disease Reporting in the Northeastern United States', *JAMA Network Open*, vol. 3, no. 3, article no. e200319, 2020.

10: Every Inch of Sand

232 'My perception drew back into my head ...': 'Depersonalisation Disorder: NHS Treatment', UK Hansard, vol. 656, debated Tuesday 12 March 2019, <hansard.parliament.uk/commons/2019-03-12/debates/B4368A54-BAF2-4732-92D1-5CA441527DA3/DepersonalisationDisorderNHSTreatment>.

233 'I fell in love with her courage ...': Fitzgerald, F.S. & Fitzgerald, Z., *Dear Scott, Dearest Zelda*, Bryer, J.R. & Barks, C.W., eds, New York: Scribner, 2019, p. 32.

Acknowledgements

The seed for this book began when my editor at the *Washington Post*, Kathy Lally, commissioned an article about my depersonalisation in July 2019 and gave me the courage to expand it. Kathy's close attention to my story and her willingness to amplify it was essential in keeping the early fire going. The process I underwent in writing the piece helped me see that *When Nothing Feels Real* could be much more than simply my own story. It could offer a window into the illness itself and be a testament to those of us living with it. I am sorry these pages will never be enough to convey the desolation at the heart of the illness. But I tried, I really tried. Forgive me for the gaps.

Alexandra Payne and Justin Wolfers, my brilliant publishers, led an extraordinary team at Murdoch Books. I am grateful to them for coordinating the remarkable talents of Nicola Young, George Saad and Kristy Allen. Thank you to Jane Morrow for her commitment to my story and to Sue Bobbermein who has seen the book promoted with remarkable verve.

Infinite thanks to my agents, Lou Johnson and Jeanne Ryckmans. From our first meeting they understood my vision and embraced it with the kind of zeal and gusto every writer dreams about. Thank you for the trust and the hard yards and for making me feel like there is a home for me among the snodgrass and bottlebrush.

I am extremely grateful to Elaine Hunter, a specialist and ambassador for depersonalisation, who met with me to speak about the illness and how it alters the lives of so many. Her work over the years has vastly improved awareness and treatment for patients. She has helped countless lives, including my own.

I wish to thank generous readers of my work over the years: Bonnie Nadell, Elinor Cleghorn, Cynthia Ozick, Eleanor Jackson, Mick Jackson, Lauren Hall, Clarissa Sebag-Montefiore, Helen Oyeyemi, Vivianne Schwarz, Rachel Yuen-Collingridge, Jessica Kean, the composer Brett Dean, and the late librettist Amanda Holden – who gave me much needed critical attention.

I have worked with many great newspaper editors over the years and want to especially thank Lindsay Duguid, who commissioned my first book review for the *TLS* and assured me I had a knack for it; and Boris Dralyuk, a tireless champion of belletrists and works in translation.

Everything belongs to my teachers, who are always with me: Anne Ferran for her early support and belief in my promise, Simone Douglas for showing me the equal beauty in clarity and abstraction, Marko Daniel for helping me see that the mess is sometimes just mess, the late Mark Cousins for his deep commitment to the student essay and for introducing me to Nietzsche's *Writings from the Late Notebooks*, and Steven Connor who convinced me that speaking in metaphors is sometimes clumsy but ultimately leads to a richer view of reality – and life.

The instruction of Tom McCarthy during the beginning of my PhD was a welcome challenge, one I sorely needed. His class on 'The Other 9/11' – Chile's military coup of September 11, 1973 – opened my eyes to history's parallels, contradictions and mirrors. I thank him for uprooting my narrative preconceptions and for his contrarian spirit.

My heartfelt thanks to Julie Byrne for her album *Not Even Happiness*, whose songs offered pure mental transport at the most despairing of times. From my listening post on a grey sofa, I travelled to the fields of Colorado, Kansas and Arkansas, then watched rain fall in empty freight yards of the Pacific Northwest.

ACKNOWLEDGEMENTS

For their friendship, I thank Niall Anderson, Kari Lancaster, Alex Massouras, Jessica Berenbeim, Cameron Wilson, Libby Bailey, Lesley M.M. Blume, Tessa Boer-Mah, Noah Charney, James Charney, Dean Mason, June Sirawatcharin, Roop Sandhu and Candace Colomac.

To my family: my life belongs to you.

Thank you to the many doctors and nurses who've cared for me over the years. You span countries, clinics and seasons. Without your knowledge, service and resilience, I wouldn't be here. Even the bad doctors – the smug and the illiterate – taught me something: those with a stethoscope can be just as lost in this life.

During the course of writing this book, there were many, many occasions when I steered my ship onto the rocks. The fog was, at times, impossibly thick, and the darkness always came too early. My wife Laura not only helped me rebuild and repair the ship but did so with encouragement, grace and good song. She removed the broken shells from my feet, one by one. Often she would say, softly, 'Stand up. It's time now.' I carry those words. They are written on my bones. My love, eternal heart, this book wouldn't be alive without you. See you in Rome – and in the waters off Nielsen Park.

Finally, to each reader, it is you who complete this. It is you.